TEACHING

&

LEARNING

IN MEDICAL PRACTICE

Edited by

J.W. Rodney Peyton

TD BSc MSc(Educ) MD FRCS(Ed,Eng & I) FRCP(Lond)
Consultant Surgeon

1998 MANTICORE EUROPE LIMITED

First published in Great Britain in 1998 by Manticore Europe Limited,
Silver Birches, Heronsgate Rickmansworth, Herts. WD3 5DN

British Library Cataloguing in Publication Data

A CIP record for this book is available from the British Library

ISBN 1 900887 00 2

*The publisher is grateful to the Royal College of Surgeons of England
for providing the front cover photograph of its lecture theatre, and to
Northwick Park and St. Marks NHS Trust for providing
the other photographs in the front cover collage.*

Printed and bound in Great Britain by Biddles Ltd., Guildford

CONTRIBUTORS

MR RODNEY PEYTON — *TD BSc MSc(Educ) MD FRCS(Ed, Eng & I) FRCP(Lond)*

Mr Peyton is a consultant in General Surgery and Trauma at South Tyrone Hospital, Dungannon, Northern Ireland. His interest in education developed while he was the General Surgical Representative on the Advanced Trauma Life Support Committee (ATLS) Programme of which he was a founder member in the UK and Ireland. He subsequently acquired a degree in Medical Education, as part of which, he set up the first multi-disciplinary Medical/Paramedical Teacher Instructor course for hospital doctors, GP tutors and Dental tutors in Northern Ireland.

Having instigated the 'Training the Trainers' course for the College and other institutions, he is now a Tutor in the Education Department of the Royal College of Surgeons of England and has run courses throughout the UK, Europe and the Far East.

Mr Peyton conceived, set up and runs intensive instructional courses in laparoscopic surgery. He also teaches courses on surgery in the Middle East. He was a member of a team from the Royal College of Surgeons of England to set up and train the trauma service for the Falkland Islands.

In 1982, Mr Peyton was awarded the TD (Territorial Decoration) with two bars as a trauma instructor with the RAMC. During the Gulf War, Mr Peyton was a senior trauma instructor to the Allied Forces teaching medical management to staff in the UK, Europe and Cyprus.

In addition to his extensive teaching experience, Mr Peyton has lectured widely, has published many papers and contributed to a number of books on a variety of subjects including trauma, surgical procedures and education.

MS LYNNE ALLERY — *BA(Hons) MA*

Ms Allery is Senior Lecturer in Medical Education of the School of Postgraduate and Dental Education at the University of Wales College of Medicine. Appointed to the position in 1994, she is responsible for overseeing teaching and researching activities and provides educational expertise to the schools, institutes and departments of the University of Wales. She took the lead in designing, directing and teaching the first taught Mastership in Medical Education in the UK.

Ms Allery's academic background includes education and psychology and she has undertaken a number of educational consultancies both within the UK and internationally. She acts as referee for Medical Education, Medical Teacher and The British Journal of General Practice and is a member of ASME and AMEE.

PROFESSOR COLIN COLES — *BSc MA PhD*

Professor Coles holds a personal chair in Medical Education at the Institute of Health and Community Studies at Bournemouth University. He has a background in biological sciences, psychology and education, and previously founded the medical education unit at the University of Southampton Medical School. His current work combines developing postgraduate and continuing medical education in the South and West region of the NHS with an academic interest in professional education and the development of professional judgement.

He is a member of the British Medical Association's Medical Education Board, the Standing Committee of Postgraduate Medical and Dental Education, and the Chief Medical Officer's Academic Forum. He has published widely in medical and multi-professional education.

PROFESSOR DUNCAN HARRIS — *BSc(Hons) MSc PhD Cert Ed*

Professor Harris is Emeritus Professor of Education, Brunel University and was formerly Head of the Education Department and Dean of the Faculty of Education and Design at Brunel University.

Professor Harris was the first educator for the ATLS in the UK and was initiator of ALS and ALSG Instructor courses. He was joint initiator of Training the Trainers course at the Royal College of Surgeons of England and has had similar roles in the Republic of Ireland.

Professor Harris has authored and co-authored over 80 papers and 16 books, most of which relate to evaluation and learning.

DR BRIAN JOLLY — *BSc MA(Ed) PhD*

Dr Jolly is Director of the Medical Education Unit at the University of Leeds Medical School. He is interested in all aspects of medical education, in particular, clinical teaching, skills training, curriculum evaluation and the assessment of clinical competence.

In 1978, Dr Jolly successfully applied for the first grant in the UK for the development of a medical MSc by distance learning. Since then he has worked on many educational programmes, developing teaching resources and styles, including student centred education and community-based medical education, and has worked on teaching courses for doctors for over 10 years.

He was awarded a PhD for work on clinical teaching by the University of Maastricht, a centre of excellence for medical education. He was recently invited to be the Secretary of State for Education's representative and a founder member of the General Osteopathic Council. Dr Jolly has written and lectured extensively on all aspects of medical education.

RALPH MORRISON — *MEd*

Mr Morrison was educated at St John's College York, The Royal Military Academy, Sandhurst and the University of Bath. He is a Training Development Consultant who has specialised in the management, design and delivery of training and has worked both in the UK and Canada. He is a member of the Education Faculty for courses organised by the Royal College of Surgeons of England.

MRS LYNNE PEYTON — *TD BSSc MSc CQSW*

Lynne Peyton is Assistant Director of Social Services (Family & Child Care) with the Southern Health & Social Services Board in Northern Ireland.

She graduated from Queens University Belfast, in 1974 and qualified in Social Work in 1977. She has extensive experience of providing both child care and mental health services including a year with the Family and Children's Service in Virginia, USA. After more than ten years in operational management she moved to her present position and now leads a multi-disciplinary team with responsibility for planning and commissioning child care, maternal health and child health services.

Lynne has a long standing interest in multi-disciplinary training and has been instrumental in the design and delivery of a number of highly successful courses, predominantly in the area of child protection.

MIKE WALKER — *Cert Ed BSc MA*

Mike Walker is a senior lecturer in Medical Education in the School of Medicine at Imperial College of Science, Technology and Medicine, London. He has responsibility for research and staff development with particular reference to the new, problem-based undergraduate curriculum. He has been involved with medical education for the past twelve years at first with GP's and for the past four years with hospital doctors.

He has just completed a two-year study of the training of junior surgeons on the cardiothoracic department of a London teaching hospital and is currently engaged on the Department of Health survey of Calman reforms. Over the past two years he has taught on more than 25 Training the Trainers courses for the Royal College of Surgeons of England as well as ALS Instructor courses for the Resuscitation Council (UK) for whom he is the Educational Advisor. He has published widely on a range of medical education issues.

TABLE OF CONTENTS

ACKNOWLEDGEMENT

I SHOULD LIKE TO ACKNOWLEDGE and thank my colleagues who have contributed and provided their support for this book.

Their knowledge and interest in medical education has enabled me to produce a book with a clarity and depth of understanding which would otherwise not have been possible.

Also, a special thank you to Cherith Cowan for the many hours which she dedicated to putting this manuscript together.

J.W. RODNEY PEYTON

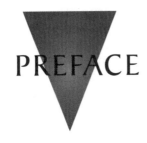

PREFACE

RODNEY PEYTON

'Practice without theory is blind
Theory without practice is sterile'

VLADIMIR LENIN (1870-1924)

TEACHING AND LEARNING within the medical profession has been undergoing fundamental change everywhere. Although written from the UK perspective, this book's contents are equally valid and applicable in many other countries that are either undergoing or planning such changes in the future. *Teaching & Learning in Medical Practice* is specifically aimed at practitioners who are engaged in both undergraduate and postgraduate education. Make no mistake, this present era of rapid scientific and technological advance means that all professionals are engaged in a continuing process of professional development. Such growth requires a learning process, and most learning requires teaching. The concepts and techniques discussed in this book apply equally to hospital-based medicine and general practice, as well as to a wider circle including dentists and other health care professionals.

When research is undertaken, there must be a basic understanding of the rules governing the selection of the research question, the research design, statistics and methods of presentation of the results. Similarly, those who teach must have a clear understanding of the principles of adult learning and motivation. By adding such an understanding to an individual's wealth of experience in teaching, learning can only be enhanced.

The aim of medical education is to produce self-motivated practitioners who continually learn and develop throughout their career. To this end, it is important to understand that those in training should not be spoon-fed, but helped to have minds capable of searching out and evaluating information that they can, where relevant, absorb into everyday practice. Teachers at this level therefore take on the role of learning process facilitators.

Most medical teaching is an everyday activity that has to be fitted in with busy clinical commitments. In recognition of the competing demands of the role of a teacher and other aspects of professional life, this text combines theory and practice in a concise manner, firmly rooted in the clinical context. Teaching must be effective in its outcomes, and at the same time represent as efficient as possible use of professional time.

This is therefore an intensely practical guide, split into two sections. Part one covers the theoretical aspects of teaching in some depth. Each chapter ends with a section describing how the theory can be put into action and a bibliography is included for those who wish to pursue some aspects in greater depth. Part two deals with a number of practical teaching situations such as on the wards, in theatre, in out-patients including general practice consultations, in small group teaching and also in the more formal settings of lectures. These chapters have a very practical orientation and are not referenced since they are based on the theoretical chapters, which precede them and also reflect the extensive personal experience of the various contributors.

All the authors are well known educators in the UK and have a keen interest in the development of medical education. Their hope is that the following pages will contribute to an increased understanding of the basic principles of education which, when applied to different teaching situations, will render the whole educational process more satisfying for the teacher as well as the learner.

THE THEORY

'Practice without theory is blind…'

The first eight chapters concentrate on the theoretical basis of teaching in the medical context. The objective is to enhance the learning process by adding an understanding of the basic principles of how adults learn and how they are motivated by the teacher's wealth of teaching and learning experience. They are equally valid to those who actively teach at the moment or wish to be involved in teaching in the future.

The theory is firmly rooted in the clinical context and each chapter suggests ways in which the information may be put to immediate use. The first chapter deals with the cycles of learning and motivation, followed by four key chapters dealing with the basic principles of adult education including methods of assessing trainees and the giving of constructive feedback. Chapters six and seven deal with course and curriculum design as well as methods of evaluating them. Chapter eight discusses the role of the educational supervisor in detail and suggests ways of making it more effective.

CHAPTER 1
The Learning Cycle

RODNEY PEYTON

INTRODUCTION

WHILE MOST doctors regard teaching as an intrinsic part of their occupation, few have had the opportunity to study teaching techniques, much less the chance to reflect on such a thing as their teaching practice.

Of course, everyone wants to be thought a good, rather than a bad teacher. After all, every doctor can remember those who stood out as such during their training. The bad ones often seem more memorable than the good.

Part of the problem is that Senior staff is used to autonomy in both clinical practice and teaching. This means that they rarely have the opportunity to receive constructive feedback to help them develop and grow in their teaching practice in the same way as properly constituted audit meetings and conferences can help medical practice. Twenty years experience as a teacher may actually reflect two years of growth in the beginning when they were particularly keen to teach and eighteen years of stagnation as their interests developed in other directions.

This chapter considers the teacher's role, and how it has altered over the last few years as a more professional approach to medical education developed. It then discusses two fundamental concepts, the cyclical nature of the learning process and the essential steps in the development of competence. Both are basic to understanding how adults learn.

TEACHING METHODS

Historically, medicine has been taught rather didactically with a prolongation of the teacher-centred learning processes, common in primary and secondary levels of education, throughout university and into the years of clinical practice. This fitted with the traditional British apprenticeship style training with a master/pupil relationship between teacher and the learner. Such modes of teaching tend to be handed down from one generation to another.

14 While authoritarian teaching methods may be comfortable for those who are insecure in their ability to handle discussion and debate on particular topics, they may also mask deficiencies in the teacher's knowledge base. Unfortunately, in the long term, authoritarian teaching tends to lead to a state of dependency on the learner's part and is not a good model for professional development.

Learners should not be seen simply as receptacles for information. They should be encouraged to seek out and reflect on new knowledge in the light of their own experience and be able to decide whether to integrate it into practice.

The teacher, then, must be an active facilitator taking responsibility for maximising the learning process by creating episodes in which it can occur. The teaching process has to do with all those surrounding environmental and interpersonal relationship events that produce a behavioural change in the learner. There is no one correct method of teaching. It is a dynamic interactive process. The skill is in knowing when to vary the input.

A heavily teacher-centred approach may perhaps be most appropriate in the early phase of learning when the knowledge base is weak and skills are limited. Later, a more learner-centred approach can be adopted as experience builds. It is a matter of knowing not just what to teach but when and how to teach it. This requires knowledge of a range of techniques and an understanding of which to use when. Thus, a wide variety of skills is required to provide education in its truest sense, 'to lead out'. The objective is to help the learners become independent practitioners committed to life long learning.

The professionalization of medical teaching requires utilisation of the basic principles of adult education in the particular context of medical practice. This theme will be further developed in chapter two. If doctors can appreciate, in practical terms, how adults learn, then they will also understand how to improve their teaching.

THE BASIS OF LEARNING

Most animals learn by serendipity – that is, they respond to stimuli. Over time they build up responses that grow into patterns of behaviour. Humans differ from animals in that they can consciously choose to learn and seek out ways of doing so. Conversely, they can choose not to learn. Learning is therefore a voluntary activity with motivation as the key. The absolute core skill of a teacher is to nurture and promote motivation, giving timely and supportive feedback and encouraging learners to reflect on any new input in the context of their work practice.

Why then do learners tolerate teachers who are inclined to be rude and cause embarrassment or humiliation? Motivation is again the key. Whilst it is true adults tend to move towards pleasure and away from pain such as embarrassment, one of the classic features of adult behaviour is the ability to defer pleasure if the perceived longer term gain is worthwhile. Motivating factors may be the achievement of a particular knowledge base or skill, success in exams or perhaps simply gaining a good reference! In practice, along with the acquisition of knowledge and skill, comes attitude development. This is considerably influenced by role modelling and helps explain how poor teaching behaviour can be perpetuated. In primary and secondary education settings, bullying tactics have long been condemned and action taken to stamp them out. Yet, in some professions, including medicine, such methods persist because they are accepted as necessary evils. In the longer term this can be entirely counterproductive. Once learners become independent practitioners, they are less likely to voluntarily re-enter teacher/learner situations, which they remember as negative and frustrating.

THE NATURE OF CHANGE IN MEDICINE

Medical practice is changing rapidly. Keeping up to date with knowledge and skills has never been more vital. Doctors find themselves on a lifelong roller coaster of teaching and learning. One day they may be experts in a particular field where they function as a teacher or facilitator for others, the next they may be forced back into the learner's role by change of circumstances such as the introduction of a new surgical technique. This is well illustrated by the manner in which laparoscopic cholecystectomy was introduced into general surgery. Although this change was indeed revolutionary, some had difficulty understanding that they needed to undergo a formal training process before carrying out the procedure. Failure to train resulted in some very serious, well-documented and highly publicised consequences for their patients.

Medical practice is evolving with less reliance on a particular individual's knowledge base or skill but rather on a team approach. These teams involve many different branches of medicine. There are representatives of the nursing profession and professions allied to medicine such as laboratory work, physiotherapy and social work, all of which can have a direct impact on the patient's health. Team working, then, is more prevalent than ever before and, given the complexity of modern medicine, this trend is liable to continue. Doctors must therefore be prepared to teach and to learn, not only within their own profession but also across disciplines.

THE TEACHER/LEARNER INTERACTION

The hallmark of a great teacher is the intense desire to have someone learn. Learning implies some process of change in the individual, whether it is in terms of knowledge base (or increased understanding), skills or attitude. Knowledge of itself has no power unless it is employed appropriately in the clinical context. When knowledge has to be put into action, confidence in both the knowledge itself and the ability to apply it successfully is vital. Like motivation, confidence can be damaged or even destroyed by inappropriate feedback.

There is a tendency to maximise the number of learners and minimise the number of teachers, treating the teaching/learning process as a kind of production line. This interferes markedly with the communication between teacher and learner, decreasing motivation for both, and can produce a very superficial type of learning. Frequently, the end result is simply the acquisition of facts to pass an examination. Once the goal is reached these are often quickly forgotten.

Adult learners respond best when treated as individuals and so the educational process needs to be capable of looking at each person's particular wants and needs. These may not necessarily be the same. The learner has to be allowed or guided to reflect on the pertinent issues, a vital step to aligning wants and needs. This synergy is basic to motivation, and the closer they are, the more efficient the learning. The teacher must therefore enable this process by becoming learner-centred, taking time to view the process from the learner's perspective.

16

THE LEARNING CYCLE

One of the hallmarks of senior members of any profession is their ability to practice on the basis of previous experience, that is by pattern recognition. Sometimes it proves difficult for them to remember when they had to learn from first principles and all of the steps involved.

There are four basic stages in the process to achieve mastery in a subject or with a technique.

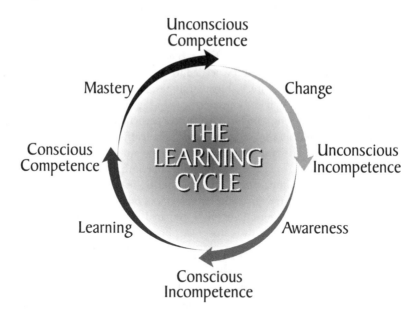

Fig. 1 THE LEARNING CYCLE

The first stage begins when knowledge or a technique comes to notice, for instance when watching an operation being carried out or a knot being tied. The learners do not actually know all the steps that have to be carried out, but paradoxically they may feel quite capable of carrying out the procedure! It is rather reminiscent of discussing football tactics from the comfort of an armchair! *They are unconsciously incompetent.*

If they try to carry out the procedure themselves and realise it is perhaps not as easy as it appeared, they become *consciously incompetent* and, providing the motivation is high enough, try to learn all the steps involved. Once they understand and can carry out the various steps then they become *consciously competent*. They still have to think about the procedure but, given time, can carry it out satisfactorily. With practice they then enter the fourth stage wherein, having mastery of the technique, they become *unconsciously competent*, implying that they can carry out the procedure without consciously having to think about it. The procedure becomes routine.

There can be a considerable gap between doing something quickly and efficiently as a master and the more laborious pace the student has to maintain during the learning process in order to get anywhere near an understanding or achievement of the same goal.

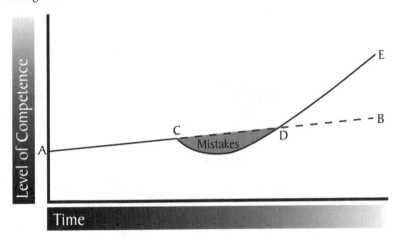

Fig. 2 THE DEVELOPMENT OF COMPETENCE

This learning process is diagramatically outlined in figure two. The present state of knowledge is represented by point A. If no new learning occurs, there may be some increase in competence over time due to experience as suggested by the line A - B. The process is routine, the practitioner is *unconsciously competent*. At point C, a new methodology is introduced. A decision is made either to learn or to reject, in the latter case the line continues as before to point B.

If the decision is to acquire the new knowledge or skill, then learning is required. The practitioner becomes *consciously incompetent* and assumes the role of trainee. During this phase, efficiency is reduced and the period is characterised by mistakes. The greater the change, the more likely that mistakes will occur. The trainee, however senior, will feel some discomfort and awkwardness and requires support and guidance. It should be emphasised that mistakes are a natural consequence and should be anticipated as the trainee learns to cope with the new situation. The trainer must allow for this by providing a supportive environment for the learning but at the same time taking responsibility for any safety issues, particularly if patients are involved. Further, it is vital that learners are encouraged to reflect on the reasons why mistakes have occurred, and to consider the implications for future practice.

Given time, which may vary widely between individuals, and the nature of the learning task, the new competency will develop and the trainee becomes *consciously competent*. Support can then be gradually withdrawn. When the new learning is appropriate, then at point D the level of competency would surpass that which would otherwise have been present and improve with continuing experience to point E. This time the trainee returns to a state of *unconscious competence*, and by definition, to independence as a practitioner, thereby completing the cycle.

18

CAPACITY TO LEARN OR TEACH

The level of existing knowledge and the learners' previous experience have obvious implications for their ability to integrate new knowledge or skills. The capacity of individuals to retain and integrate information depends not only on innate intelligence and experience, but also on whether or not they are tired or distracted, perhaps by work or social problems. Misconceptions and mistakes are apt to occur. Accordingly, arranging teaching episodes at the end of the working day (or worse still on Friday afternoon or Saturday morning) is not conducive to efficient learning. Neither is it true for efficient teaching. Teachers in the professions have many other service commitments of which, usually, teaching is only a small part. Most wish teaching to be as efficient as possible to avoid compromising clinical activity or their own life outside work.

A common misconception is that teachers must increase the amount of teaching in order for learners to increase their amount of learning. The good news on this front is that there is no such direct association and learning will be enhanced more by improving the quality, nature and relevance of the teaching than by an increase in its volume. Improvement is brought about by relating theory to practice and by considering the basic principles of how adults learn each time a teaching episode takes place. A short period of reflection afterwards, either individually or with a peer group, will help the teacher to continue to grow and develop his teaching practice, thereby developing more effective and efficient methods of helping the learner.

Finally, not everyone wishes to teach and there should be no obligation to do so. However, those who teach well should be acknowledged. Indeed, they must be if their motivation is to be sustained. Indeed, those with teaching aptitude should be regarded as highly as those professionals recognised for their superior clinical expertise or contributions to research. There are many constraints including time, workload, finance or environment which can interfere with the teaching process. However, when a good teacher really wants to teach and feels valued for doing so, most of these constraints can be overcome or considerably mitigated.

CONCLUSION

It is said that one retains five per cent of what is heard, ten per cent of what is seen and up to ninety per cent of knowledge that is put into action. When adding any new skills to established techniques, whether it be teaching or even an operative procedure, levels of competence appear to diminish before they improve. This is because time must be spent thinking and reflecting on the new skills at the level of conscious competence or even conscious incompetence.

With perseverance, the new skill or technique becomes fully assimilated and, if it is appropriate for the individual, will lead to greater levels of performance. Some elements of the theory and practice outlined in the subsequent chapters will be second nature to those who teach regularly, other parts will be new or at least offer a different slant on old ideas. The following pages will contribute to an increased understanding of the basic principles of education which, when applied to different teaching situations, will render the whole educational process more satisfying for the teacher as well as the learner.

SUGGESTED FURTHER READING

Brookfield, S.D. (1986) – Understanding and facilitating Adult Learning. Open University Press, Buckingham

Brown, G. & Atkins, M. (1988) – Effective Teaching in Higher Education. Routledge, London

Knowles, M. (1990) – The Adult Learner–A Neglected Species. Gulf Publishing Company, Houston, Texas

Newble, D. & Cannon, R. (1987) – A Handbook for Medical Teachers. MTP Press Limited, Lancaster

Oxley, J. (1997) – Multi-professional Working and Learning: Sharing the educational challenge. SCOPME, London

Ramsden, P. (1992) – Learning to Teach in Higher Education. Routledge, London

Rodgers, A. (1986) – Teaching Adults. Open University Press, Buckingham

CHAPTER 2
Principles of Adult Education

MIKE WALKER & DUNCAN HARRIS

INTRODUCTION

THIS CHAPTER BEGINS by looking at, and contrasting education for children and adults. From these considerations it identifies practical problems in the adult learning context. For instance, it is usually part-time, constrained by professional and domestic commitments, and undertaken from varying levels of confidence and competence. The chapter suggests responses to these variations followed by a more in-depth analysis of how adults learn from experience. It discusses development of expertise, features of professional knowledge and, finally, the nature of expert knowledge and conceptualisation and implications for adult learning.

CHILDHOOD LEARNING RECONSIDERED

To talk about teaching and learning somehow still invokes memories of teachers, schools and pupils. We may have enjoyed or suffered school. We may have been good at our lessons or not. There is one thing, however, that all pupils do successfully learn; they learn about teaching and learning. Very few of them leave school without knowing exactly what is involved in teaching and learning. This is part of the unwritten curriculum they will carry with them into their adult lives.

Dickens nicely caricatured the assumptions upon which childhood learning is founded in 1854. In *Hard Times* he showed Thomas Gradgrind presiding over the Coketown School where its pupils 'the little pitchers before him...were to be filled so full of facts'. Gradgrind reminds the schoolmaster to 'Teach these boys and girls nothing but facts. Facts alone are wanted in life'. Actually, they learn rather more than just facts. For instance, there is a new girl in the class, whom Mr Gradgrind addresses:

'Girl number twenty,' said Mr Gradgrind, squarely pointing with his square forefinger, 'I don't know that girl. Who is that girl?'

'Sissy Jupe, sir,' explained number twenty, blushing, standing up and curtsying.

'Sissy is not a name,' said Mr Gradgrind. 'Don't call yourself Sissy. Call yourself Cecilia.'

'It's father as calls me Sissy, sir,' returned the young girl in a trembling voice, and with another curtsy.

'Then he has no business to do it,' said Mr Gradgrind. 'Tell him he mustn't. Cecilia Jupe. Let me see. What is your father?'

'He belongs to the horse-riding, if you please, sir.'

Mr Gradgrind frowned, and waved off the objectionable calling with his hand.

'We don't want to know anything about that, here. You mustn't tell us about that, here. Your father breaks horses, don't he?'

'If you please, sir, when they can get any to break, they do break horses in the ring, sir.'

'You mustn't tell us about the ring, here. Very well, then. Describe your father as a horse-breaker. He doctors sick horses, I dare say?'

'Oh, yes, sir.'

'Very well, then. He is a veterinary surgeon, a farrier and horse-breaker. Give me your definition of a horse.'

(Sissy Jupe thrown into the greatest alarm by this demand.)

'Girl number twenty unable to define a horse!' said Mr Gradgrind, for the general behoof of all the little pitchers. 'Girl number twenty possessed of no facts, in reference to one of the commonest of animals! Some boy's definition of a horse.'...

'Bitzer,' said Thomas Gradgrind. 'Your definition of a horse.'

'Quadruped. Graminivorous. Forty teeth, namely twenty-four grinders, four eye-teeth, and twelve incisive. Sheds coat in the spring; in marshy countries, sheds hoofs, too. Hoofs hard, but requiring to be shod with iron. Age known by marks in mouth.' Thus (and much more) Bitzer.

'Now girl number twenty,' said Mr Gradgrind. 'You know what a horse is.'

What Sissy will have learned from this exchange will have little to do with horses and much to do with the fact that teachers and examiners have knowledge that pupils must acquire. She will have learned that only their knowledge 'counts' and that knowledge gained from experience is discounted. Of course, this is meant to have happened a long time ago, it is fictional and it relates to children rather than adults.

However, a recent study of medical students and their progress through medical school describes an introductory lecture in which the new students were advised that:

> At school you were taught with the object of getting here as medical students, against stiff competition. Now the onus is much more on you: you are now adults and so it is extremely difficult to force you to learn.

There is the expectation here of a different approach to teaching and learning, one that recognises the learners' adult status and an attendant readiness to accept responsibility for their own learning. However, towards the end of the students' second year, a follow-up study observed that:

> More than half their time during the first two years was spent in lectures. Most took place within the medical school, in an old-fashioned tiered lecture theatre dating from the 1930s. The whole year attended lectures together, peering down at blackboard and lecturer and scribbling frantically for an hour at a time.

No doubt, these students were engaged in the gathering of facts from which they would emerge Bitzer-like able to give definitions on request. The problem with this approach to teaching undergraduate students is that it seems to operate with the same notions of teaching and learning that characterise school teaching from its inception in the mid-nineteenth century. These medical students seem to have remained 'little pitchers to be filled'. How else might it be?

The traditional view is that adults learn in a way that is quite distinct from the way children learn. Thus, the teachers' role and relationship with the learner must shift. The principle characteristics of adult learning are that:

- adult learning is purposeful
- adults are voluntary participants in learning
- adults require active participation in learning
- adults need clear goals and objectives to be set
- adults need feedback
- adults need to be reflective.

These points are elaborated below, but can be read more fully elsewhere. (See suggested texts such at Brookfield and Knowles at the end of the chapter.) They must be actively addressed in any teaching/learning situation. If they are ignored, they become obstacles and barriers to continued growth and development.

ADULT LEARNING CHARACTERISTICS

Adult Learning is Purposeful

For an understanding of adult learning we should first look at how children learn. For the child pupil the purpose of schooling may be unclear. Explanations given in terms of preparation for life, of obtaining a good job, of entering university or of becoming a good citizen hold little relevance for a twelve-year-old. Indeed, twelve-year-olds probably have alternative versions of the 'purpose of schooling'. Even so, most will take it on trust that one day the purpose of their studies will be revealed to them.

Adult students are different. With the hard won autonomy that comes with growing up and the need to earn a living, they are far less willing to take value and relevance on trust. Adults are much more likely to engage in learning only when they have a specific purpose in mind. This does not preclude learning as a means of enjoyment or for some intrinsic value, but it does suggest they approach learning with a purpose in mind. For instance – 'When I retire I want to live in France and I want to be confident and articulate in French by then' or 'This will help me gain promotion,' or 'Drawing these graphs by hand is tedious, I need to learn how to do it on the computer'. What this sense of purpose implies is that they approach whatever teaching is provided, in a particular way. Adults examine the provision of courses, lectures, seminars, or tutorials and ask 'How does this help me?' What is more, they are selective in their uptake and want to negotiate adjustments that tailor the official provision to fit their needs. Failure to anticipate this and to respond appropriately can result in less than effective teaching.

The illustration below is taken from a study of a course for General Practitioners. The course tutor, L, has invited an expert, JR, to lecture to the group on questionnaire design. However, most of the group, including D have already designed theirs and begun piloting them. At this stage, they are looking for specific guidance rather than general principles.

JR arrives and L introduces him with a small portrait, the research he has done, his current work. It is the portrait of an expert.

For the benefit of the group JR conducts a tutorial with D. He is trying to show, from within his social science paradigm, how questionnaires are meant to work. D's answers to his questions are prompted by a detailed knowledge of the issues of her practice. What she wants to find out about are those issues and the work she has already done in designing a questionnaire. He questions her from one perspective, she answers from another. This is not the answer needed to take further his exposition of the rules of questionnaire design. But this is not the question she needed to help her confront the issues of her project. It's an uneasy negotiation. Now the group are invited to contribute, which they do in volume. JR seems to have opted out, he is sorting through his papers. This discussion ranges around the course members own projects and their problems. JR says nothing.

One could claim that there is a conflict in perspectives between the academic and the practitioner. On the other hand, it is also possible to see that D has a purpose and is pursuing it, whilst JR is thwarted in pursuit of his. *If it was his purpose to teach questionnaire design theory, then he has failed.* An alternative approach for JR would have been to collect and classify all of the problems the group were having with their questionnaires and deal with each class of problems by giving practical guidelines plus an explanation of the problem and it's solution. In this way he could have moved from their problems/perspectives to his, aligning their wants with their needs as perceived by both JR and L.

Adults are Voluntary Participants

Some are on courses, or attempting to study, simply because they were told to do it for their own and the organisation's benefit. In such cases individuals may be reluctant learners. They are not the norm. A vast majority of adults seek education because they believe it will help them to achieve a particular purpose. This implies a number of things. Firstly, unlike in schools there is not the time-consuming problem of managing learners' behaviour, secondly, teachers of adults can usually rely on an initial reservoir of goodwill and, thirdly, learners will contribute and participate enthusiastically in teaching sessions. All of these positive attributes are contingent upon the teacher's ability to further the learner's purpose. The prime importance of motivation in adult learning cannot be overemphasised. It is discussed in greater detail in Chapter Three.

Adults Require Meaning and Relevance

Some years ago one of the authors (MW) addressed a group of experienced school-teachers on disruptive pupils in the classroom. He began by describing the work of an obscure 19th century French scholar, but was quite unprepared for the waves of hostility and resentment coming from his audience during the first ten minutes of the talk. However, once the scholar's principles had been clarified and the audience had had the opportunity to apply them to classroom management problems, the atmosphere became much more positive and productive. Unlike children, adults will not wait for years to see whether the knowledge they acquire from teachers will be of value in everyday life. Of course, the seminar could have been structured differently. It would have been better to begin with principles and applications and progressed to origins and derivations. Indeed some of those who were most disgruntled at the outset subsequently asked for more details of the scholar's life and work.

An important feature of this anecdote is that although the audience became cross, some more than others, the antagonism was general. Adults value the opportunity for study and have high expectations related to their purpose. They know such study comes at some cost and time, and in spite of professional and domestic pressures. When they sense disregard for their expectations and purpose, they become upset.

The illustration below is taken from the diary of James, a General Practitioner taking an MSc course in General Practice. As part of this course he took a module on Adult Learning, which seems to have had on him an effect similar to that which my seminar had on its audience some years before.

Today I became angry...it is not something I often experience, but today I did in the small group session. (My tutor) was obviously uncomfortable and angry - he doesn't hide his feelings. I am a GP - that is my job, I'm doing an MSc in general practice yet it seems that any attempt to relate this learning to my work is disallowed. I often feel that we have lost sight of our role as GPs - that the substance of the sessions bears little relationship to what we actually do. If I can't relate what I am doing on a Wednesday to what I do the rest of the week I can't feel justified in continuing the course with all the costs to myself, to my family and partners.

This particular quotation could be used to illustrate so many facets of adult learning but here it is used to show a learner's determination to maintain relevance to purpose - and the consequences when this is blocked.

Adults Require Active Involvement in Learning

Some years ago Paul Willis published an influential study of a group of disaffected boys in a secondary comprehensive school. (See suggested further reading.) The group referred to themselves as 'the lads' and, by contrast, to conformist pupils as 'earoles'.

Willis explains that, The term 'earole' itself connotes the passivity and absurdity of the school conformists for the lads. It seems that they are always listening, never *doing*: never animated with their own internal life, but formless in rigid reception'.

In opposition to both the earoles and authority 'the lads' seemed to take control of their own destiny, often thwarting teachers and school authorities for their own amusement. They were active in their own learning and learned a great deal although little of it was on the school curriculum. Significantly, they regarded themselves as more mature than other pupils. It was this supposed maturity that may have been the cause of their continuing conflict with teachers (although this is not the argument Willis presents). However, it does suggest, that once we go beyond being prepared to sit and listen there is an urge to get on with doing the learning. To be clear here, active involvement may consist of getting up and doing things like practising psychomotor skills, being involved in an open, small group discussion, collecting data of one kind or another, or finally, it may mean simply sitting in a lecture actively listening and reflecting.

Books deliver information; human beings communicate knowledge accentuated with ideas, opinions and emotions. Lectures can, and should be, so constructed and delivered that the audience is mentally (and perhaps verbally) involved, challenged, entertained, worked and absorbed throughout. Delivering this type of lecture is difficult even if the learners' general purpose is known. (This purpose may be obvious. If you have a class full of trainee nurses for example, they must want to qualify otherwise they wouldn't be here.)

Despite this, meanings and relevance may not be immediately obvious to the learners and would have to be guessed or estimated on the basis of experience. In an open discussion with a small group there is undoubtedly a much greater opportunity to ascertain relevance and discover meaning. This is one reason why small group discussions are often more effective than lectures with adults. The same argument would apply to workshops, skill stations, role-plays, simulations, and projects.

Adults Need Clear Goals and Objectives to be Set

To enhance learning potential set clear goals and objectives. First let us look at objectives. These specify what should be learned and allow us to assess whether or not learning has taken place. Goals are equally important and differ from objectives in small but crucial ways. They usually specify time periods and thus mark out a sequence of events or a number of stages en route to the overall aim of the educational process. For formal courses, at least, course organisers and examining boards and the like, usually set goals in advance. For individuals who have been away from formal learning for some time or who lack confidence, short-term goals would be most appropriate. An example would be 'for our meeting next Wednesday you will need to read…'. More experienced and more confident learners might need goals specified in terms of weeks or months rather than days.

However, objectives are usually negotiated between teacher and learners. Objectives help to organise the learner and can be reset to match changing needs. What is important in negotiating the objective is that the learner as well as the teacher agrees that it is achievable. 'Achievable' here implies that learners believe they not only have the intellectual capacity to complete the tasks, but they have the opportunity, the agreement and understanding of colleagues and family, the requisite material resources and whatever else it might take to achieve completion. This all adds up to what is sometimes referred to as the learners 'capacity to learn'. Note that this is described not only in terms of their intellectual function, but also in terms of their resources, including time constraints.

Tiredness and worry can significantly impair intellectual capacity and therefore the ability to learn. This simple fact has considerable practical implications in the organisation of teaching episodes either after a full days work or in running an 'educational' event from early morning to late evening.

Goals, and specifically objectives, therefore have to take into account and need to be adjusted to fit, changes in the learner's circumstances and context. Should they be unrealistic and unachievable a sense of failure results. However, when they are realistic, no matter how small or short term they are, a sense of achievement is still produced when they are attained.

Recently, goal setting has become more popular and slightly more formal, through the notion of educational contracts. Here the learner meets with the supervisor, tutor or mentor on a regular basis. At the first meeting they discuss the learner's wants and needs and the needs of the organisation. Goals are identified followed by a learning plan with specified objectives. This learning plan should include details of each party's responsibilities.

The tutor agrees, for instance, to provide certain forms of formal and informal tuition, access to experiential learning, opportunity for reflection and feedback, whilst the learner agrees to attend meetings, undertake preparatory work, write assignments and reports and so on. When each party is satisfied, they will sign the contract. Contracts can be renewed on a weekly or monthly basis. The learning contract has many advantages. Firstly, it brings system and order into a situation where previously there was none, hence its increasing popularity in the training of junior hospital staff. Secondly, it can match the needs of the organisation with those of the individual. Thirdly, if goals and objectives are well set then completion can bring a sense of satisfaction to both parties. Each party will have the opportunity to assess and provide feedback on the degree to which they have been achieved and the contract fulfilled.

Setting goals and objectives therefore profoundly influences the direction and outcome of learning. Thus, they are an essential skill, and will be discussed in greater detail in Chapter Four.

Adults Need Feedback

There is a common-sense obviousness about feedback. Any learning task from tying shoelaces, improving a golf swing or performing Hamlet is made easier if there is immediate information on the initial attempts. Often this will come from personal observation. If the shoelaces come undone then the attempts were unsuccessful. For a more complex task it may be necessary to enlist the help of someone more expert to describe and analyse the performance and offer remedial advice. Giving such advice is a skill in its own right. There are those, even within the ranks of professional educators, who see this task as being concerned exclusively with the identification of 'mistakes'. After all, they argue, it is the mistakes that need to be corrected!

On this view, feedback is a listing of everything that went wrong albeit with the more enlightened tutors providing suggestions for improvement. Giving feedback should not be an end in itself, but rather an integral part of the learning process. To facilitate this a more positive approach should be adopted based on the application of four enquiries:

28

- Ask the learner what went well or what she was particularly happy with in the performance.
- Ask other learners what they did well.
- Ask the learner how the performance could be improved.
- Ask the other learners what could be improved.

The tutor then sums up the specific points of good practice and particular suggestions for improvement. This approach to feedback has the merit of highlighting and rewarding what was done well, probably 90% to 95% of the performance, and making positive suggestions for improvement in the remaining 5% to 10% of the end performance.

This very powerful method of critiquing a performance merits further review. Asking the learner and others involved what went well should not be seen as a brief social nicety to be got out of the way before the real meat of the discussion. Positive reinforcement of good practice helps to ensure its continuance both in the learner being critiqued and in others partaking in the session. They may hear indicators of good performance they had not thought of themselves and think to incorporate them into their own practice. It is important to realise that the learner may lack insight and feel happy with those elements of his performance that the tutor may regard as less than satisfactory and require correction. In this case the appropriate area can be revisited during the 'suggestions for improvement'.

The third enquiry is specifically 'what could be improved'. It is important that this is not simply a list of negatives. It should be looked at in a positive light with a view to making future performance better. There is always a tendency for both learner and peer group to offer a long list of what they feel went wrong and then look to the tutor for improvements. The overall aim is to produce professionals who are self-analysing and thus continually striving to improve themselves.

The tutor must force them to think along those lines and to come up as far as possible with their own solutions. This does not mean that important issues should not be raised. If necessary, the tutor must steer the conversation in the appropriate direction. However, as far as possible, it is important the tutor asks learners to come up with their own suggestions for improvement before volunteering his own comments. Finally, the tutor should summarise the session following the rule of threes. One of the group, or better still the learner himself, lists at least three specific positive points and two or three specific points for improvement. Note that it is important that this is regarded as a summary of the session and should only include points raised in the discussion, not new issues.

Feedback, then, is important for two reasons. Firstly, it gives the learner and the group feedback about how well they are performing. It thus enables them to adjust their efforts. The more immediate the feedback the better they are able to make the adjustment. Secondly, having made such adjustments, positive feedback acts as a reward, reinforcing those actions and ensures that they are repeated. For both these reasons, positive and immediate feedback acts as a powerful extrinsic motivation for the learner.

Thus far we have considered formal feedback, responses to lectures or presentations, comments upon written work etc. Much feedback, however, is of an informal kind. In everyday situations it may not be necessary to always give the appropriate signals through expression, posture or gesture, and of course it might be more convenient for us as teachers if all learners were sufficiently robust not be affected by our comments. Mind you, then we should probably regard them as arrogant and impervious to advice. The truth is that most in a learning situation develop the ability to disguise their sensitivities, but this does not mean that they are insensitive.

Professionals and teachers bear a responsibility to assist those they teach to actually learn. They should be aware that, even informal feedback such as smiling, scowling, grunting, slouching, and alertness can all effect the learner. The process may easily be damaged by careless or insensitive informal responses.

Adults Need to be Reflective

Individuals reflect on their studies by themselves, with a mentor, or with their peers. This reflection involves reviewing recent experience and estimating how it contributes to, or hinders, their attainment of objectives or goals.

For instance, how can incoherent experiences, mistakes, opportunities, or critical moments help them?

For the learner to find experience useful, this dissection and evaluation is crucial. To this end, opportunity for reflection must be part of any learning dependent on on-the-job training, apprenticeship or the supposed result of 'experience'. Opportunity for reflection is perhaps most important of all in cases where experiential learning is seen as a substitute for or an addition to formal teaching. In such cases, reflection may be built into appraisal, audit, or continual professional development systems.

Reflection, in its broadest sense, is usually achieved through verbal exchanges, but it can also be experienced through contemplation, in written form and by discussion. In the written form learners keep diaries for recording both significant events and their responses to them. The significance of events is judged by whether or not they promoted learning. Thus, some days may pass when little has happened to promote any fresh insights. Below is an extract from a diary written by a learner on a formal course:

I was disappointed with myself because the session I ran with Helen was a flop. I had thought that my enthusiasm for the topic would be enough, but it wasn't. They were bored. Why didn't I stop and ask them? I didn't, I just carried on. This has made me feel separate from the group and critical of them.

In this instance, the learner gained a number of insights into teaching and learning. Although, it may be impossible to demonstrate this point conclusively, a good case can be made that if this learner had simply mulled over her 'session' rather than writing it down in an organised way in her diary, her realisations about it would have been less powerful and penetrating. Thinking about events is useful, writing about them or discussing them with others is more useful.

The focus for discussion is often 'critical incidents'. These are incidents that have, in some way, challenged the individual's attitudes, skills, or relationships. The opportunity to reflect upon critical incidents, to put them into perspective, gain support and feedback from peers and others and to learn from the experience is particularly important for novice learners. For someone at the beginning of his or her training, there is much to learn and there are many mistakes to make.

Below is an illustration taken from a group of student nurses discussing critical incidents:

> It was past dinner time. I said to him 'Are you alright?' He said, 'I feel terrible,' then he started to bleed again. I thought, 'I can't deal with this'. I ran out and said, 'Will somebody help me with this?' I ran back to him – he'd been sick everywhere. There was such a lot of it. I should have pulled the emergency bell. I didn't do it. Then everyone came charging in and started saying, 'Do this, do that'. It really did shock me. I realised then he was seriously ill but no one had said, 'This man's really ill'. I just thought he was alright.

Clearly, the incident had impact upon this student. Unfortunately, what we do not have here are her fellow students responses and the realisations to which she came as a result of the discussion. One would hope that there might have been some exploration of the distinction between 'alright' and 'really ill' which would have informed future practice.

Reflecting with others prevents us following our natural tendency to dwell on what we did badly and ignore what went well. As was suggested in relation to feedback, recognising and accepting what went well is an important motivational element.

THE CONTEXT OF ADULT LEARNING

Thus far the discussion of adult learning has dwelt on its principles. This is as it should be since these principles provide not only the educational goals but also the practical guidelines for contributing to adult learning. This section examines some of the more practical issues arising from attempts to implement these principles.

Formal education usually ceases at 16 or 18 years of age or for those who, in increasing numbers, are going on to higher education it may continue until the age of 24 or 25 years. In this way, adults will have spent anywhere between 11 and 20 years in a formal education system based upon the passive, receptive approach of childhood education discussed earlier. This has important implications. Their conceptions of teaching and learning are essentially those of the passive pupil. They will expect a standardised curriculum taught by subject experts in a formal way.

They will expect to be the recipients of knowledge, to be told what to study, to have their performance assessed, and to be told what they have done wrong. It seems that, regardless of their experiences since the end of their formal education, and regardless of learning that they will have undoubtedly achieved in the intervening period, when they return to formal education they will become, once again, dependent upon their teachers. They will expect to be taught as they have always been taught. For teachers of adults this is the first, and perhaps most difficult, hurdle to clear.

Because adults engage in learning voluntarily and because that learning is rendered meaningful through its relationship to individual purpose and experience, over-dependency upon a teacher is inappropriate. Indeed, Knowles argues that the point at which people take responsibility for their own growth and development is the point at which they become psychologically an adult. The first problem for the teacher of adults is how to decrease this dependency and enable learners to take responsibility for their own learning. Once this happens, adults become liberated and able to use their enormous innate potential for self-development. This process may take some time, but it begins with relationships.

In the traditional model, the teacher acquires status by virtue of being an authority on some particular subject. By virtue of having to organise the learning of reluctant and unruly learners, the teacher must also be in authority. On these two counts, the learner mode is one of deference. Unfortunately, on returning to formal education, adults carry this baggage of deference with them. Even when they may be painfully aware that what is provided for them is not meeting their needs they will not assume responsibility for changing matters themselves. Indeed, when evaluating courses dissatisfied adults often criticise teachers for not being sufficiently 'teacherish'.

The route away from dependency begins with defining and updating this relationship to one of mutual respect. Learning is worthwhile. This means that, by definition, all involved in the process are doing something worthwhile. They deserve other learners respect. The fact that some will have spent longer learning and been more successful than others is unimportant. What matters is that at any one point in time the effort to learn, at whatever level, is deserving of respect.

In practical terms, this implies that learners efforts, verbal or written, need to be accepted and their contribution positively evaluated. It also implies that where appropriate, teachers should use the same process to share and jointly evaluate their efforts with learners. This exchange of learning experiences, successful or otherwise between 'teacher' and 'learner' helps to reduce deference and to promote the notion that between learners there are no status distinctions. In their turn, learners should not simply rely on the teacher but should place greater value on their own efforts.

There is a second advantage to this shift in relationships. It allows the learner's experiences in day-to-day matters to be brought into the learning context. As was noted earlier, traditional modes of teaching tend to exclude personal experience. For adults, however, personal experience is usually an integral part of their purpose, an element in their motivation and a rich source of insights into personal development. The question then becomes 'how can personal experience best be used to facilitate learning?'

In the first instance, this may mean the teacher identifying with the learner precisely what has prompted him or her to undertake learning at this moment. In most cases, the motive will be pragmatic and probably job related. The learner needs to acquire a qualification, to work more effectively in order to change occupations or gain promotion and so on.

Hence, the learner's purpose is to satisfy a need within his everyday experience. To achieve this end, it will be important for both teacher and learner to use the learner's work based experience. Of course, individuals may opt to learn about topics such as the history of military battles, wildlife of the Kalahari or Egyptian hieroglyphics, that are entirely unrelated to their everyday experience. But even these subjects may be purposefully chosen. The learner, for instance, may have taken a holiday in Egypt and decided to return this year.

Once the learner's primary concerns have been identified, they can be introduced into the tutorial or group discussion. This is not to suggest that seminars or tutorials should be reduced to a string of anecdotes. Rather, the intention is to build conceptual bridges between academic and experiential knowledge. In the example given earlier, James was doing just this, although his tutor sought to deny him this opportunity.

James had also recognised similarities between his own efforts to make sense of an unknown discipline (Adult Learning) and those of his patients trying to make sense of the medical consultation. He saw in his patients attempts to understand their illness and the medical process, a reflection of his own efforts to make sense of the theories of adult learning. James' reading of educational ideas and his reflection upon his own practice led to, what was for him, a genuinely new insight - that he and his patients are 'co-learners'.

James's tutors should have been delighted that he was making such connections and that he was drawing upon his experience in such a productive way. To begin with, learners may not be able to offer such insights. Therefore, the responsibility for demonstrating such connections will fall to the teacher. The process of identifying links and how this is done will, in itself, be the subject of discussion and analysis. Identifying how and why links are made advances understanding of the learning process. Moreover, it also validates experiential knowledge as part of the learning process and thus establishes the adult as an independent learner.

Thus far, we have established that to reduce dependency we need mutual respect between learner and teacher in order to demonstrate the legitimacy of experiential knowledge and its potential contribution to learning. In addition, we need to recognise how adult and childhood learning differ. Childrens roles are less diverse, their responsibilities fewer and of course their purposes less well defined. Ideally, adults require individually tailored tuition that fits in with their intellectual needs and professional and domestic commitments.

Negotiated Education and the Adult Context

Once we begin to take the individual learner's purpose seriously, and we begin to use experiential knowledge as a learning resource, then the notion of providing a standard course for a homogeneous audience becomes much more problematic. As individuals and as a group, learners will want to negotiate over the form and content of their educational experience in order to ensure the closest fit with their needs.

For children and most undergraduates, education is a full-time activity. For most adults it must be accommodated alongside a full-time job and, in all probability, time consuming domestic commitments. The problem with domestic and professional responsibilities is that their requirements are unpredictable and uneven. They lurch from making heavy demands upon the individual's time, energy and emotional resources into periods of relative ease. The individual's educational efforts are likely to follow this erratic pattern because they have little option in placing the needs of their family and job before their educational needs.

For the teacher this poses yet another problem. With the traditional approach to teaching adults or anyone else for that matter, the integrity of the course and the course arrangements come first. Those who enrol on the course agree to comply with these arrangements, to attend classes, to undertake directed study, to prepare assessments and submit them on time. Any deviation from this may result in the individual's failure to satisfactorily complete the course. While individual teachers have usually allowed some latitude, the onus has always been upon the learner to provide satisfactory evidence to explain non-attendance or lateness in submitting work.

33

According to this view, the teacher's responsibility is simply to deliver the course. Those learners with sufficient ability and determination will pass, others will not. If one adopts the principles of adult learning then these arguments become questionable. At very least, the teachers role changes from provider of academic content to learning process facilitator. In practice this is likely to mean spending time in counselling and supporting individuals at the expense of providing curriculum content. It is likely to mean continually helping to set (or revise) goals in response to changes in the learner's circumstances, accepting work at unscheduled times, providing additional tuition in non-specified areas, being available and easy to contact outside teaching hours and so on. A shift from traditional to adult learning then poses problems for teachers as well as learners.

Experiential Learning

The previous section addressed some of the common issues in teaching adults. In this section the nature of adult learning and in particular, experiential learning will be examined in more detail. The basis for an explanation of experiential learning is usually presented as a cycle:

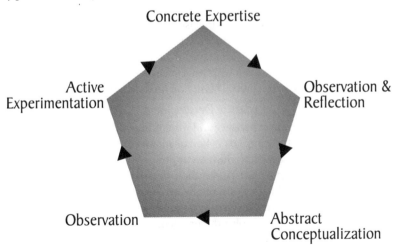

Fig. 1 SCHON'S EXPERIENTIAL LEARNING CYCLE

The premise here is familiar; learning occurs through reflection on practice. This particular notion is also associated with Schon (see suggested further reading) and his seminal work on the 'reflective practitioner'. Schon argues that:

> The process (of reflection on action) spirals through stages of appreciation (of an issue) and active re-appreciation. The unique and uncertain situation comes to be understood through the attemp to change it and changed through the attempt to understand it.

Schon's attempt to describe the relationship between work, knowledge of work, and our understanding of work has been highly influential. However, it seems to lack a basic element. To correct this omission an alternative formulation of the learning cycle might be:

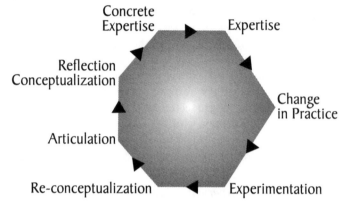

Fig. 2 EXPANDED EXPERIENTIAL LEARNING CYCLE

What is added here is the notion of articulation. Articulation is necessary in order to sequence reflections and to make them accessible to others. In presenting our reflections to others, we invite feedback, endorsements, challenge, enhancement and the possibility of reformulation. In this we intensify our perceptions of experience and increase our ability to express them. These are precisely the arguments used in advocating discussion as an appropriate technique for adult learning.

Thus far it has been suggested that we learn from experience, and that at some stage we shift from being novices to experts. This notion needs to be explored in more detail.

Expertise Development

We continue to learn from experience and we continue to accumulate experience. However, at some point, there appears to be a qualitative change in the nature of our experiences, at least in those aspects which occupy must of our time, such as our occupation. At some stage, we gain mastery over the process, the tools and the knowledge, skills and perceptions by which we earn our living. We become experts.

Clearly, all degrees of expertise involve the notion of having mastery over the means by which we resolve issues and solve the problems confronting us daily. Mastery involves being able to use our knowledge and skills to a higher purpose. We might take the learner driver as an illustration of this idea. The learner driver is much occupied with the controls of the vehicle, being conscious of how and when to depress the clutch, use the gear lever or apply the brakes. The expert driver, however, has mastery over these processes and focuses attention instead upon safely negotiating the traffic. The expert driver is able to use the vehicle for a higher purpose – commuting, racing, touring – and so on. Occupational learning can be viewed in the same way with similar distinctions between the learner or novice and the expert.

The term occupational knowledge is used here quite deliberately instead of the more usual 'professional knowledge'. Having done that, one engages in an unavoidable argument. When using the term 'professional knowledge' one suggests that the process of acquiring expertise and expert knowledge is confined to those occupations having 'professional status'. Of course this is not the case. If it were, one would be left with two approaches to adult learning, one catering for the professional and one for the rest. Experience and logic tell one that this is not the case and therefore the argument must be confronted before going any further.

Professional Knowledge

Some occupations claim that they have special distinguishing traits setting them apart from other occupations and allowing them to claim professional status. These traits usually include:

- Esoteric knowledge derived from long and rigorous training
- Autonomy of practice within the workplace
- A governing body that controls standards and admissions
- A code of ethics which places the interests of the client and the community before self-interests.

As a justification for the special status of professional knowledge there are problems with this formulation. For instance, it has been argued that such traits may not be a description of actual behaviour but merely claims made by occupations to secure professional status and benefits. Equally, they may be regarded as 'market strategies' enabling those in such occupations to seek to increase their services market value. It may be argued that long and rigorous training with time spent in reflection and conceptualisation sets them apart from those in non-professions.

However in that model profession, medicine, report after report has lamented the total lack of time for reflection in training. Hence, it seems that the distinction between professional expertise and any other form of expertise is a highly dubious one. Indeed, it may be akin to regarding Bitzer's knowledge of horses as superior to that of Sissy Jupe. Nevertheless in what follows the writers often refer to professional knowledge or expertise, although it will be left to the reader to decide whether their ideas have application beyond the narrow confines of 'the professions'.

Expert Knowledge

The learner driver will again serve as an illustration of novice learning. The learner driver begins by learning the rules, (check mirror, manoeuvre, check mirror) but for the expert the rules have been absorbed into a general approach. This argument may be taken further in looking at the nature of professional expertise. It would appear that experts do not apply their knowledge through a formal systematic analysis based upon rules and clear cut factual propositions. On the contrary, he argues that,

This is how novices, still dominated by recent book-learning set about taking their first faltering steps into the practical work before they have built up the forms of proficiency and expertise which will enable them to do without it. In contrast, the fully proficient professional worker's knowledge is no longer in the form of rules and facts, but consists of rough guidelines, elliptical maxims, long range goals which determine priorities and a repertoire of typical examples which are available to invoke as precedents.

At this level, expert knowledge has become almost intuitive, situationally specific and context bound. It will also become more difficult to articulate hence the notion of indeterminate knowledge which characterises occupations by the ratio of their technicality to their indeterminacy. Technicality refers to those aspects of work where rules and procedures can be made explicit where techniques can be analysed and explained. By contrast determinacy refers to aspects of work evolving through practice. These are tacit and unique and that cannot easily be formulated into rules or recipes. The acquisition of indeterminate knowledge requires 'a lengthy period of induction into the arcane knowledge of the occupation'. Indeterminate knowledge is then the core of expertise and not surprisingly it arises from experience which is the heart of the matter and should be the basis of all theory. [Winter; see suggested further reading.]

The question then becomes, 'What is it about the work experience that provides the opportunity to become expert?' What do we do with the raw material of experience in order for it to become expert knowledge? One argument is that through reflection we are able to type and classify our experiences. This allows unique incidents to be recognised as conforming to a particular type. In other words, we learn to generalise about our experience, and generalisation is the first step toward being able to develop concepts or abstractions.

Abstraction in this context, means that process by which practitioners refine their understanding and increase their conceptual grasp of their work through reflection. The development of abstraction and conceptualisation can be illustrated by a recent description of nurse education by one of the authors in which differences between the perceptions of ward work held by senior nurses and student nurses were highlighted.

The students often felt overwhelmed by the volume of tasks facing them. They found it difficult to organise, systematise or prioritise the mass of details they perceived. For instance, they could follow the instructions they had been given for taking individual readings, but unlike senior nurses they could not see them as an integral part of the systematic monitoring or the patient's shifting state of health.

When caring for patients, the student saw a patient whose hair need combing but was unable to categorise it, as the senior nurses did, as an aspect of appearance, a component of self and a contributor to morale and well being. In other words, the student nurses had a much lower level of ability to conceptualise their daily work.

Through conceptualisation we perceive objects, events or processes as having essential similarities that may be differentiated into classes, groups or patterns. Classification and differentiation is the basis upon which we build ideas into hierarchies network systems, model and theories. The teacher of adults, then, will assist the learner in moving from rules to concepts, models, and theories.

CONCLUSION

It will always be easier for teachers of adults to assume, like Mr Gradgrind, that learners are 'possessed of no facts'. In this case, all that teachers have to do is pour in the facts. Indeed, many learners want to take the role of empty pitchers, and will expect to be filled with bright new knowledge.

Hopefully, the ideas presented above will have demonstrated that the reality of the matter not only differs from this view but is also considerably more complex. Learners have different levels of experience and vary in the extent to which they can convert experience to higher level concepts. They vary in levels of self confidence and the ease with which they can decrease their dependency upon teachers. And, of course, their commitment to learning will vary with changes in their domestic and professional circumstances. For these reasons, the traditional course is bound to be somewhat limited in its effectiveness. A more effective approach to the teaching of adults can be assembled from the theoretical and practical considerations outlined here.

37

PUTTING THIS CHAPTER INTO ACTION

Along with some of the possible responses the main issues discussed in this chapter are summarised below.

1. Socialisation

    Adult learners often retain traditional views of teaching and learning derived from their experiences as pupils and students.

    Response

    Explore with the learners the assumptions about teaching and learning inherent in the childhood model. Compare these assumptions with their individual and group needs. Identify educational arrangements that accommodate their present needs.

2. Deference and Dependency

    Learners tend to be deferential towards and dependent upon the 'expert' teacher. This inhibits their learning.

    Response

    Show, and help to develop, mutual respect for co-learners. Recognise and respond positively to learning efforts. Share your own learning efforts, including difficulties and failures with the learners. Where possible, use open discussion techniques and encourage peer evaluation.

3. Experiential Learning

    Whilst recognising the relevance of their day to day experiences for themselves, learners may be reluctant to see this as a part of real learning.

    Response

    Identify ways in which we learn from experience and explore good and bad learning experiences. Identify similarities in the learning process at work and on the course. Apply concepts introduced on the course to non-course experiences. Be prepared to modify concepts, models or theories to gain a better fit with experience. Compare course based knowledge with experiential knowledge.

4. Individualised Learning

Because of their professional, domestic and other commitments the effort which adults can expend on learning is variable and unpredictable.

Response

Be flexible and accept that course arrangements may have to be in a continual state of negotiation and modification according to need. Require more of the curriculum content to be covered by the learners in their own time and at their own pace. Devote more time to counselling, goal setting and supportive activities. Discuss the problems of part- time study with the group, encourage the sharing of practical solutions to past problems, and highlight the advantages of collaborative study.

5. Provision of Feedback

Adults require feedback on their efforts so that they can maintain the process of reflection and self-improvement.

Response

The technique of providing positive feedback using the four enquiries should become second nature. Remember the aim is to produce learners who will wish to self-correct wherever possible. This will not just involve thinking out problems but coming up with their own solutions and ways of implementing them. Show the group this method of critiquing and encourage members to run their own feedback sessions along these lines.

6. The Teacher's Role

A shift to the principles of Adult Learning may require just as much re-thinking on the part of the teacher as it does for the learner.

Response

Read and become familiar with the ideas and concepts. Initiate small changes and discuss results with learners. Share the experience with colleagues. Review your existing teaching and identify which elements conform to adult learning principles and which do not. Prioritise areas for change, monitor the outcomes and compare with previous efforts. Reflect upon practice.

SUGGESTED FURTHER READING

Beard, R. & Hartley, J. (1984) – Teaching and Learning in Higher Education. Paul Chapman Publishing, London

Brookfield, S.D. (1986) – Understanding & Facilitating Adult Learning. Open University Press, Buckingham

Knowles, M.S. (1990) – The Adult Learner, A Neglected Species. Gulf Publishing Company, Houston

Ramsden, P. (1992) – Learning to Teach in Higher Education. Routledge, London

Rodgers, A. (1992) – Teaching Adults. Open University Press, Buckingham

Schon, D.A. (1990) – Educating the Reflective Practitioner: Towards a New Design for Teaching and Learning. Jossey Bass, San Francisco

Walkin, L. (1993) – Teaching & Learning in Further & Adult Education. Stanley Thornes (Publishing) Ltd., Cheltenham

Winter, R. (1991) – Outline of a General Theory of Professional Competencies: The ASSET Programme of Anglia Polytechnic and Essex County Council Social Services, Chelmsford

Willis, P. (1977) – Learning to Labour. How Working Class Kids get Working Class Jobs. Saxon House, Farnborough

CHAPTER 3
Motivation in Teaching and Learning

RALPH MORRISON

INTRODUCTION

THIS CHAPTER begins with a review of approaches to what motivates people and how the process occurs. The four basic drives motivating students to learn are outlined and ten ways to increase classroom motivation are suggested.

The Intrinsic Drive

Can teachers motivate students or are they only motivated by the need for something (status, affection or achievement)? Are students motivated by a lack of something? Is it a mixture of both? Because the word is used ambiguously does it mean that we are unsure what is really meant by it?

Teachers must understand student motivation. They must grasp the fact that most want to learn. At the same time, teachers must also realise that motivation cannot be counted on and that the most dedicated student can be put off by an uninterested teacher with poor presentation skills, badly designed surroundings, poor material or even tiredness and worry. Somehow, students must be persuaded to actively involve themselves in the learning process. Although, it may be stimulated, activated and encouraged by the teacher the necessary drive must come from within.

Quite simply, students are best motivated when they want to do something. Motivation covers all the reasons making a student to act. These include positive rewards and recognition and negative reasons such as fear of teachers or exams. Motivation caused by avoidance of a consequence is, however, liable to lead to superficial learning behaviours. Learned material is quickly forgotten when the fear is removed. If teachers do not know how to encourage, maintain and develop their students' motivation then their task becomes almost impossible. Teachers must be aware that motivation is easily damaged if they are indifferent to students' needs, respond negatively to their efforts or make assessments and give feedback without explanation.

Such activities cause resentment or anger and prevent learning. Problems with motivation only arise when students are forced to learn things they do not want to know or that seem inappropriate. Under such circumstances, there is a temptation to rely on negative motivators such as fear of failure or punishment with the predictable consequences outlined above. Therefore, the teacher should make understanding those factors affecting motivation a priority.

If teachers can understand and predict student motivation they have the opportunity to influence them by changing the components of that motivational process. There is no guaranteed formula of motivation but there is now a better understanding of the complex process of how a student reaches decisions on the achievement of his or her ambitions and on time, energy and talent use. However, even if there is no general formula, understanding the process helps the teacher to explain some of the problems and difficulty students might have with the learning process.

A student's performance on any task is determined by three major factors. Firstly, he or she must have the intellectual ability to carry out the task in question. Secondly, the right learning environment must be provided so the student can develop intellectual abilities or competence. Thirdly, the student must be motivated to complete the task. The relationship between performance and motivation can therefore be expressed as:

Performance = Intellectual ability & competence x Motivation.

The teacher must be aware that there is an interaction between intellectual ability and motivation. Thus, if a student has little ability, even a very high level of motivation will still produce a poor performance. However, if there is a reasonable amount of ability, the effect of even small increases in motivation will produce a better performance.

WHAT IS MOTIVATION?

The most important concept underlying any learning experience is motivation. A student is motivated when he or she wants to do something. A motive is not quite the same as an incentive. For instance, a student may be inspired or made enthusiastic by an incentive, his or her main motive for wanting to do something may be avoidance of punishment. Thus, motivation can be positive or negative. It covers all the reasons underlying a person's actions. It is probably the single most powerful determinant of an individual's willingness to learn.

Motivation is a difficult concept to understand, but can be defined as 'that within the individual, rather than without, which incites him or her to action'. In other words, motivation is a drive state that produces action from which satisfaction is derived. The key is in knowing how to use this drive state to enhance the learning experience.

Motivation theory attempts to explain why individuals take some actions and reject others. In observing a collection of students performing the same task it will be seen that their performance varies. One obvious reason for this is the different levels of skill amongst the students. The performance of a particular task, however, depends not only on skill but also on desire. Motivation refers to this latter requirement and involves the needs, drives and goals which make up the major determinants of behaviour. There are four major assumptions that can be made:

1. Man is goal seeking. Behaviour is caused by attempts to achieve specific goals. These goals, in turn, are related to an individual's satisfaction of particular needs. At any given time, a person's thoughts and actions are an outgrowth of their perceived needs and goals.
2. Needs and goals, as well as the actions flowing from them are closely related to such factors as an individual's self-image, status, group affiliations, and perceptions of the environment.
3. The relationship between needs and goals on the one hand and thoughts and actions on the other, is extremely complex and unstable. The same needs may stimulate different behaviour in different people and different behaviour in the same person at different times. Also, similar behaviour can be based on the operation of different needs.
4. Every individual has a large number of diverse needs, but at any given time only a small subset of these needs is subject to conscious action. This subset is determined by the individual's physiological, psychological and environmental states at that particular time.

CONTENT AND PROCESS THEORIES

Motivation theories are sometimes divided into 'content' or 'process'. Almost all theorists make assumptions about individual needs, or drives. Content theorists, such as Maslow, Alderfer, Herzberg and McLelland, describe *What* it is that motivates. On the other hand, process theorists, describe the subject process - the *How* - of motivation. They assume the existence of cognitive antecedents. This means that we learn by experience. Unsatisfactory past experiences can adversely affect our present situation. Positive prior experience of appropriately rewarded performance or skill use motivates us to perform well again. Process theorists include Vroom, Adams, Porter and Lawler.

Content Theories

MASLOW'S THEORY

It was Abraham H. Maslow who developed a motivational model based on a hierarchy of five levels of satisfaction. He viewed motivation in terms of an individual's striving for growth and sought to explain as a 'hierarchy of human needs'. People are 'wanting animals'. Maslow believed that at any given moment a person's most potent needs dominated his or her behaviour. As his or her 'lower', physiological needs are adequately satisfied, motives at a 'higher' level in the hierarchy come into play. The hierarchy is made up as follows:

1. Physical needs, for example hunger, thirst, leading to a desire for food and water
2. Security needs such as a highly anxious student may experience
3. Social needs such as friendship
4. Ego needs such as success
5. Self-actualisation needs such as a desire for self-fulfilment.

Motivation at levels four and five (often referred to as *intrinsic motivation*) is very important and should be taken into account in the planning of work related to the ultimate goal of the realisation of students' potential abilities.

According to Maslow, the five levels of needs are related to one another in a sequential fashion starting with the physiological needs at the bottom of the hierarchy and progressing upward through the other levels until self-actualisation is reached at the top. Self-actualisation implies a state in which the main drives are internal and independent of feedback or outside motivation. Satisfying needs at the lowest unfulfilled level of the hierarchy is an individual primary motivation.

When the needs at this level are adequately satisfied, the individual moves up to the next level of needs. These become dominant in determining his actions. This usually means that once a lower level need is satisfied it no longer motivates. It follows that the only needs motivating behaviour are those that are still unsatisfied.

Maslow's hierarchy suggests that as physiological needs are met, and survival and security needs satisfied, individuals may be expected to respond more effectively to respect, status, and self-actualisation rewards than to economic rewards primarily related to the satisfaction of lower-level needs.

Three important points have to be remembered about Maslow's theory:

—The hierarchy closely resembles a person's ordinary development from birth to maturity. First, the infant needs food and warmth, safety and love. As it grows, it needs to develop a reasonable self-assurance (or self-esteem). Finally, it emerges as a self-motivating adult capable of and desiring achievement.

—As they are satisfied one set of needs disappear and others emerge as motivators is an unconscious process. Once a qualification is gained one quickly forgets and denies the pleasure of attainment and starts looking towards the next qualification, status, or recognition. Lacking the attainment of this qualification makes one miserable. It is as if one has no qualifications.

—As Maslow points out, the five steps in the hierarchy are not rigid. There is a certain degree of interlock between them. It is more a matter of decreasing percentages as one ascends the steps, since most members of society are, at the same time, both partially satisfied and partially unsatisfied in all their needs.

Despite, or perhaps because of its generality, Maslow's theory can be criticised as follows:

- There is no evidence that satisfying any one need leads to predictable behaviour.
- The same need may cause different behaviour in different people.
- Behaviour is not a function of any one need therefore the theory is too simple.
- Some individuals willingly forego satisfying immediate lower-level needs in order to fulfil a longer-term, higher-level need. For example, an aspiring surgeon may endure early student 'hardship' in order to achieve career goals.

As a theory of motivation therefore, Maslow's cannot stand alone. However, he never intended that it should. As an acknowledgement of a variety of needs, and as a stimulus to further research, Maslow's theory is an important contribution to understanding human behaviour.

Other research into needs identifies similar lower-level needs categories to Maslow's. In general, research suggests that needs fall into a two-level hierarchy, with 'lower-level security needs' on the bottom and 'higher needs or wants' on the top.

HERTZBERG'S MOTIVATION-HYGIENE THEORY

However, it was Frederick Herzberg's 'Two Factor Theory' or 'Motivation Hygiene Theory' that stimulated the most interest in recent years. In this 'motivators' and 'hygiene factors' such as recognition, responsibility and the feeling of accomplishment affect individuals. To the degree that these are present in the classroom, motivation will occur and have a positive effect on learning. Hygiene factors are those primarily associated with the context of an activity. As applied to the classroom setting, examples of such factors are the teacher's instruction style, the learner's security, and classroom interpersonal relationships. When present, hygiene factors prevent dissatisfaction, but do not necessarily lead to satisfaction.

ALDERFER'S ERG THEORY

Clayton Alderfer extended both the Herzberg and, especially, the Maslow content theories of motivation. He formulated a need category model that was more in line with the existing empirical evidence and reformulated Maslow's hierarchy into three levels. Similar to Maslow and Herzberg, Alderfer believed in the value of categorising needs and that there is a basic distinction between lower-order needs and higher-order needs.

Alderfer identified three groups of core needs: Existence, relatedness, and growth. (Hence, the ERG theory). Existence needs govern survival (physiological well being). Relatedness needs stress the importance of interpersonal, social relationships. Growth needs are concerned with the individual's intrinsic desire for personal development.

In addition, Alderfer's identified both a 'need satisfaction process' and a 'need frustration regression process'. Thus, a student experiencing repeated frustration in his efforts to satisfy some higher-order needs, will place greater importance on the preceding lower level needs.

A Comparison of Content Theories

Figure 1 shows how Alderfer's groups of needs relate to the Maslow and Herzberg categories. Obviously, they are very close, but the ERG needs do not have strict lines of demarcation.

Alderfer suggested more of a continuum of needs than hierarchical levels of two factors of pre-potency needs. Unlike Maslow and Herzberg, he did not contend that a lower-level need has to be fulfilled before one of a higher-level motivates or that deprivation is the only way to activate a need. For example, under ERG theory, background or cultural environment may dictate that relatedness needs take precedence over unfulfilled existence needs and that the more growth needs are satisfied, the more intense they become.

There has not been a great deal of research on ERG theory. Although there is some evidence to counter the theory's predictive value, most contemporary analyses of work motivation support Alderfer's theory over those of Maslow and Herzberg. Overall, the ERG theory takes some of the earlier content theories' strong points but is less restrictive and limiting. However, the fact remains that most content theories do not explain the complexities of motivation. With the possible exception of the implications for instructional design of Herzberg's work, they do not readily translate to the actual practice of human resources and management.

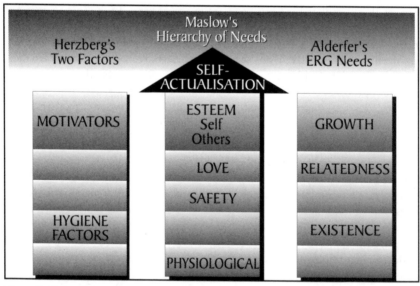

Fig. 1 THE RELATIONSHIP BETWEEN ALDERFER'S ERG NEEDS, MASLOW'S FIVE-LEVEL HIERARCHY, AND HERZBERG'S TWO-FACTOR THEORY

The Maslow, Herzberg, and Alderfer models attempt to identify specific content factors in the individual (in the case of Maslow and Alderfer) or in the environment (in the case of Herzberg) that motivate students. Although such a content approach has surface logic, is easy to understand, and can be readily translated into practice, the research evidence points out some definite limitations. There is very little research support for these models' theoretical basis and predictability. The trade-off for simplicity sacrifices true understanding of motivational complexity. However, on the positive side, the content models emphasise important content factors that were largely ignored by the human relationists. If the Alderfer model allows more flexibility, the Herzberg model is useful as an explanation for student satisfaction.

Process Theories

In attempting to explain individual motivation, Vroom, Porter, Lawler and others have advanced a number of process theories. Process theory of motivation is based on certain behaviour being produced by particular stimuli. An example of this was Pavlov's experiments with dogs salivating. It was later found that behaviour could be shaped simply to the expectation of reward or punishment.

47

Developed by Vroom in the mid-1960s, *Expectancy Theory* states that motivation depends on the following perceptions:

- That there is an expectation that an outcome will bring the desired rewards.
- The required performance is within the capability of the person.

Therefore, it is the student's personal equation, either conscious or subconscious, that determines motivated or de-motivated behaviour. The teacher's task is seen as making explicit the link as illustrated:

EFFORT ➡️ PERFORMANCE ➡️ REWARD

These factors' direct relationship achieves effective motivation. If a student considers a particular reward attractive but needing great exertion, he or she will put more effort into working towards it. At present, because it recognises that a student's behaviour is to a considerable degree influenced by that student's expectations of what will happen in the future, expectancy theory is the most influential.

Since different incentives motivate students it is difficult identifying required rewards that are within the teacher's means. Good career prospects or a good report making them possible, are obvious student motivators. However, they are unlikely to extend over a whole course. One of the most effective student motivators is the teacher's attention and recognition. In other words, letting students know their efforts are valued. The implications for teachers are:

- Teachers should make clear to students exactly what is expected.
- Students need to be confident that they have the skills and can accomplish the task.
- Students should be able to see a connection between their efforts and the rewards that they generate.
- Teachers must know their students well enough to determine what rewards the student needs and what the teacher can give.

The expectancy model focuses on the individual. Assumptions regarding individual needs and objectives are not made. A course of action will be taken if it is likely to accomplish personal goals. This emphasises the important motivation-managing link between personal and organisational objectives.

In recognising Vroom's concept, several models have been advanced. Of these the Porter and Lawler models are the most useful. According to this model, motivation is a dynamic process affected by factors both within and outside the individual and depends upon:

- The expectancy that successful performance depends on effort.
- The expectancy that reward depends on that performance.
- The value placed on that reward. (The reward will depend largely on the individual's needs as suggested by Maslow.)
- The effort that is exerted based on the personal equation.
- Whether this effort leads to accomplishing the task will depend on the student's skill, education and personality and the facilities and organisational climate provided by the teacher.

When all these factors are taken into consideration then, other things being equal, the result will be task accomplishment where successful performance is based on effort. However, the remaining question is whether the successful performance will in itself lead to satisfaction.

Successful task accomplishment offers two types of rewards: intrinsic and extrinsic. The process theories provide a much sounder theoretical explanation of motivation. Vroom's expectancy model and the extensions and Porter's and Lawler's refinements help explain important cognitive variables and their relationship to one another in the complex motivation process. The Porter-Lawler model also gives specific attention to another the important relationship, that between performance and satisfaction.

Porter and Lawler propose that performance leads to satisfaction, instead of the human relations assumption of the reverse. Growing research literature supports these expectancy models, yet conceptual and methodological problems remain. Unlike the content models, those dealing with expectancy are relatively complex and difficult to translate into actual practice.

THE MOTIVATIONAL CYCLE

From these theories it can be stated that motivation is a basic psychological process. Comprehension of it lies in the need-drive-incentive sequence, or cycle. (Figure 2.) The basic process involves needs (deficiencies), that set in motion drives (deficiencies with direction) to accomplish incentives (anything which alleviates a need and reduces a drive).

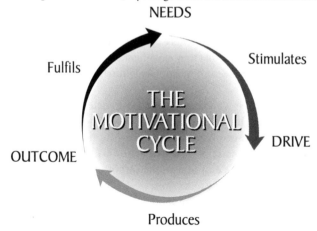

Fig. 2 THE MOTIVATIONAL CYCLE

Motivating Students

A teacher's every action stimulates some reaction from students. Therefore, there is no question of whether or not a teacher influences student motivation, the only question is whether or not it is for the good. It is important to emphasise that motivation is not something that the teacher does to his students. All the teacher can do is attempt to create an environment wherein students learn willingly or even enthusiastically. Meanwhile the teacher must remember that students will have diverse reasons for wishing to learn.

The learning process is voluntary. It is the teacher's job is to promote and maintain the desire to do it. An important task for the teacher is his or her use of power to arouse, regulate, and sustain enthusiasm for learning in the service of the lesson. Drive is the basis of classroom self-motivation and harnessing the learner's drive is of paramount importance.

Crucial as student motivation may be, it is the most important and difficult to apply successful instruction principles. Although self-motivated students exist, (intrinsic motivation), most need the teacher to motivate them to greater or lesser extent (extrinsic motivation). The teacher must make the student want to learn by actively promoting the desire to learn and once students are motivated, the teacher must maintain that desire.

Most teachers consider the presence of motivation essential to effective communication and learning. Motivation arouses, sustains and energises students; it assists in the direction of tasks; it is selective in that it helps to determine students' priorities; it assists the organising of students' activities. Tutors in higher education are well aware of the relative ease of teaching highly motivated students and of the frustrations and difficulties arising from lessons with students who, for example, see no link between their aspirations and curriculum content. The former usually exhibits behaviour calculated to assist the learning process; the latter may display a resistance, making effective learning difficult or impossible.

Student motivation may be an effective learning pre-requisite, but it is also a challenge teachers face. They must also be aware that if students regard a teaching episode as irrelevant they will not be motivated to take part in the teaching/learning process. The problem will not go away if it is merely ignored and so, the teacher must restore the student's need and drive. In all this the teacher must see the problem from the student's standpoint.

There are four basic drives that can motivate students to learn; intrinsic, extrinsic, social and achievement motivation. However, it should be noted that more than one category may dominate learner motivation at any given time.

Intrinsic Motivation

Intrinsic motivation, the most powerful of all comes from within. It is that feeling or urge that makes a student want to learn. Curiosity, inquisitiveness and a desire to meet challenges may characterise the learning set of students thus motivated. Herzberg suggested that intrinsic goals such as accomplishment and achievement are true motivators and so the relationship between these rewards and motivation is likely to be direct and strong.

A common source of intrinsic motivation is the setting of a career goal. For example, someone deciding on a career, establishes a goal. To achieve that goal, the individual has to successfully complete a course. The course may include subjects that the student must take, but may not like or understand the need for. However, to achieve a career goal, the student learns the material long enough to pass the course.

Extrinsic Motivation
(Sometimes called instrumental motivation.)

Factors (including strategies to make students learn) that are external to the individual are known as extrinsic motivation. This type of motivation is evident where students perform tasks solely because of consequences such as obtaining a reward or avoiding a reprimand. It is in total contrast to intrinsic motivation. In the face of motivation of this nature, the teacher should ensure that the task to be performed is placed in a context perceived as pleasant. There are two types of extrinsic motivators; positive and negative.

POSITIVE MOTIVATORS

Examples of positive extrinsic motivators include friendly competition between students to see who can score higher on a test. Students want approval and enjoy being successful in measuring themselves against their peers. Therefore, competition often produces strong motivation in a class of students. However, competition needs to be treated with care. The increase in motivation and self-esteem of the winners may be more than offset by the decrease in motivation and self-esteem of those who perform less well.

NEGATIVE MOTIVATORS

Negative motivators include tests, quizzes, grades, classroom questioning, and other type of standards that are set as a condition for successfully completing an activity. Negative motivators tend to produce an underlying fear or anxiety that causes the student to learn a certain amount of material in order to achieve a goal such as successfully completing a test. Invoking fear or anxiety may cause a student to learn but material retention is short-lived. The danger is that some negative motivators can be used as instruments of coercion, that is, as a means of getting students to do (learn) something they otherwise might not be inclined to do.

There is a fine line dividing positive and negative motivation. So fine is it that in many instances it is hard to draw. The teacher's intention and the student's perception is paramount. For instance, we have already seen that 'friendly competition' is a positive motivator. However, what are the effects of a competition when the extrinsic rewards are in short supply, for example, limited places on a course? The student's motivation may be the 'ignoble satisfaction of feeling that one is better than someone else'. However, in general it can be said that positive motivators are more successful in improving learning than negative motivators and enhance retention.

Social Motivation

We are social animals and gain our basic sense of identity from relationships. Students motivated thus perform tasks to please those they respect, admire, or whose opinions are important to them. Even tangible rewards are of limited significance. The reward here is non-material and is related in direct measure to the perceived relationship between the student and the person whose reinforcement activity in terms of praise or approval is considered important. Teachers must mobilise and build on these social relationships remembering the importance of teaching style and class behaviour.

Achievement Motivation

In this form of motivation students learn 'in the hope of success'. For the teacher, this is a useful concept that has some validity in the classroom when motivating students to learn. Ausubel suggests that there are three elements in motivation of this type:

- *Cognitive drive* – the learner is attempting to satisfy a perceived 'need to know';
- *Self-enhancement* – the learner is satisfying the need for self-esteem;
- *Affiliation* – the learner is seeking the approval of others.

The persistence of students to master objects and ideas suggests that they have a strong desire to achieve. This can be utilised by teachers.

PUTTING THIS CHAPTER INTO ACTION

The question all teachers strive to answer is 'How can I make a student want to learn?' The answer is that the teacher must create a learning environment that relates the student's activity to his or her needs and aspirations. In this fashion, the student develops and strengthens competence and heightens the sense of self-improvement. The teacher is the linchpin, the facilitator, and the manager of a student's learning experiences. Therefore, an understanding of student motivation is crucial for the teacher as motivation is a prerequisite for effective learning. The following ten suggestions, based on understanding motivation, should increase it in the classroom.

—*Learning depends on motivation.*

Teachers must be aware of what causes student behaviour to change into the necessary learning mode. For the student, learning involves dealing with situations. Depending upon their behaviour or response, the outcome is reward or punishment. The teacher can manipulate the perceived outcome and hence motivation to increase learning. Motivation is the most significant principle of learning. Students must be motivated to learn. Ultimately, the desire to learn must come from within. Teachers are responsible for creating the environment and conditions conducive to motivating their students. If students do not accept the need for education they will not be motivated to participate and accept and assume responsibility for their own learning.

—*Make learning interesting.*

Often teachers have to teach subjects which their students see of being no direct use to them. If teachers are to gain the student's interest and increase motivation, they must give the student a full explanation of the significance of the unacceptable subject module in terms of content, its links with the subject as a whole, and its contribution to an understanding of that subject. Short-term goals, the passing of examinations for example, must not be depreciated in any way as they are very important in the eyes of the student. Any teacher appealing to students to broaden their horizons is also likely to go unheeded.

51

Therefore, the teacher needs a positive approach to link students' long-term goals (professional competence) and short-term goals (the need for the student to expand their levels of knowledge of different subject modules). The teacher must link unacceptable subject modules with long-term goals, thus stimulating interest and increasing the students' motivation. A student who wishes to become a doctor may see no use in studying history. What the teacher needs to do is try to make connections to their interest thus making it relevant.

For instance, any study of the Crimean War might include advances in medicine and patient care made at that time. By doing this, one simply uses the basic principle that students find more interesting something that relates to them personally. Also, it goes without saying, that to increase student interest the teacher must show interest and enthusiasm. The golden rule of motivation is that teachers will never inspire others unless they are themselves inspired. Motivated teachers are competent since they believe in and like what they are teaching.

By using a variety of motivating techniques interest amongst students can be stimulated. The fatigue that accompanies boredom destroys motivation and can be avoided by a planned variety of teaching and learning techniques.

—*Ensure that the learning experience is relevant to the student.*

When preparing a teaching episode, teachers must always think in terms of student relevance. Ideally, teachers should show how relevant their lessons are to the real world and to their students' own lives. If the teacher is teaching about improvements to Public Health then they should talk about the illnesses that the students, or their parents and grandparents, have had. It is not always easy, but if successful, student motivation will be greatly enhanced.

—*Give regular feedback on performance. Let students know how well they are doing.*

It is necessary to distinguish differences in types of motivation. For instance, what is achieved through test or examination grading and motivation is quite different to what comes about through feedback in terms of appraisal of how the student actually performed during the assessment exercise. Teachers use assessment to test their students' assimilation of lesson material. What should be happening is that students should perceive it as being meant to help them in the process of learning.

Feedback, given as appraisal or 'knowledge of results', is the degree to which students get information about the effectiveness of their efforts. This is the lifeblood of learning. The basic intention of such feedback is to motivate. Having said or done something of learning significance, students want to know how it has been received. A quick response may be required if it is to modify or confirm present understanding. Feedback motivates students by rewarding them through recognition of their contribution to the class, confirmation that they are on the right track, and through identification of any additional knowledge or skill still required. In other words, effective feedback enables students to identify their strengths and weaknesses and to act on them. The teacher has the critical responsibility for developing these opportunities.

There are many forms of feedback. In its least useful form, it comes as a mark or grade. Teachers must be aware of the potentially de-motivating effect of this type of feedback. A grade for a single essay provides little information and an overall grade for a whole examination even less. Students will be uncertain about their relative performance in all subjects. Another kind of feedback the student may be given is simply the knowledge of whether they passed or failed.

Feedback becomes more useful to the student when it includes constructive comments. The teacher needs to tell the student which aspects of his performance were strong or weak and make suggestions for improvement. It is worth pointing out that feedback can also be conveyed through body language. A teacher's smile, scowl, laugh or gesture can motivate. The practicalities of giving feedback are discussed more fully in Chapter Two.

—*Reinforce the positive not the negative.*

The essence of being a good teacher is the ability to give students positive motivation enhancing feedback. The teacher must leave the student feeling confident and determined to do better next time. Teachers fail if their feedback upsets, demoralises or discourages their students. All students benefit from constructive rather than obstructive criticism.

This method of giving feedback should be done verbally. Students should be given the first opportunity to identify their own strengths and weaknesses. If teachers can persuade students to include self criticism while they are honestly and accurately assessing their own performance teachers can concentrate on confidence building measures. If teachers have established a proper learning environment this should be easy. Firstly, they must reinforce any strengths the student identifies. Then they must confirm the student's identification of any weakness. Finally, any significant points the student missed must be introduced and suggestions for improvement made.

—*Learning feeds on success.*

The desire to be successful and increase self-esteem is a powerful motivator. Thus students can derive personal satisfaction from the learning process. They generally enjoy doing what they are good at rather than what they are bad at. Success breeds success. It is odd but teachers often underestimate the effects of success and reinforcement.

If students experience success and reinforcement through praise and teacher/peer approval, their self self-confidence and self-esteem improves. This increases motivation and students' work improves. This leads to students experiencing even more success. However, if the student's sense of failure is reinforced through criticism, lack of feedback or personal satisfaction then he or she believes that the task cannot be achieved and self-confidence and self-esteem falls. Thus is student motivation eroded. Their work deteriorates and this leads to further failure. Temporary failure ought to be used by both the student and the teacher as a catalyst for a fresh attempt to overcome difficulties. Failing a test can motivate but only if students are confident in their own ability to eventually succeed. Constant failure is a huge de-motivator.

Students must know exactly what they are expected to do and how to do it. Help has to available for students if they need it. Some tasks should be straightforward and quickly achievable so all students can experience some success. Other tasks may stretch the more able. However, tasks that are either too difficult or too easy to attain do not motivate. Praise given as quickly as possible on an activity's completion reinforces success in learning. These points are crucial to motivation in most teaching situations and teachers must consider them carefully. Success should therefore be both individual and routine for all students.

—*Give students the responsibility for learning.*

It has been said that the ultimate goal of the educational system is to shift to the individual the burden of pursuing his own education. However, many students believe that in order for them to learn, all they need to do is attend classes and complete assignments and work more or less willingly. There is an expectation that learning will follow automatically. The teacher must try and make passive learners into active learners.

To do this the teacher must have the correct attitude and approach. The role is subtly changed and to encourage students to take responsibility for their own learning the teacher must become the facilitator or learning manager. Students must be encouraged to decide and negotiate their own learning needs, set their own targets, and monitor and assess their own learning.

Giving students responsibility for their own learning develops in them a self belief and autonomy rather than dependency and is important in their motivation.

—*Ensure that the right learning environment is provided.*

Motivation is not an end in itself and only benefits learning because it increases attention to the learning task, mental effort, and perseverance in the face of difficulty. If the classroom environment is distracting, students may find it difficult to achieve, despite being motivated. The physical environment is all too often ignored by the teacher and not enough attention is given to the correct (most suitable) layout of the classroom. Teachers must ensure that the physical conditions are appropriate to the particular teaching episode being taught. These may include lighting, temperature and type of furniture, as well as the position of the board, and overhead projector. Students may be distracted and difficult to motivate unless their physiological as well as psychological needs are adequately satisfied and efficient learning will not take place. The teacher has the task of creating a learning environment that relates to the learner's activity to needs and aspirations. In this way, students develop and strengthen competence. This gives them a heightened sense of self-improvement.

—*Reward good performance and discipline where necessary.*

The theory underlying 'reward and punishment' is that behaviour can be modified. Behaviour that is rewarded will occur more frequently. Behaviour that is either punished or not rewarded will occur less frequently. Student competence and mastery should be recognised by the teacher and reinforced and rewarded by praise and appreciation. In this way a student gains status and a sense of achievement. Rewards must be appropriate for individual students. What is appropriate to one student may not be to another. Teachers should link effort and performance with reward in the eyes of the student.

However, teachers will often face the problem of the student who, although well able to, does not demonstrate learning. This may simply take the form of failing a classroom test through lack of revision. Students need to know that there are consequences for not learning and that they are liable to be unpleasant. Otherwise negative reinforcement may be produced if the student comes to believe that something they dislike and decide not to learn can simply be dismissed without any sanction.

—*Goals should translate into specific objectives and students must have opportunities to satisfy their personal goals.*

Performance is increased when teachers set specific objectives with the learner following on a course's more general goals. This improvement can be enhanced if appropriate targets are agreed for each stage towards the objective. Teachers must also ensure that short-term achievements are understood in relation to long-term goals. If these goals and objectives are developed with the students themselves, they are likely to be more motivating. The setting of personal goals is valuable in that participation may lead to acceptance of more difficult goals. All must be achievable. Students who, for whatever reason, fail to achieve agreed goals will become de-motivated.

SUGGESTED FURTHER READING

Adair, J. (1990) - Understanding Motivation. Talbot Adair, Guildford

Cooper, C.L. & Makin, P. (1984) - Psychology for Managers. Macmillan Publishers Ltd., Basingstoke

Child, D. (1986) - Psychology and the Teacher. Cassell Education Ltd., London

Curzan, L.B. (1990) - Teaching in Further Education. Cassell Education Ltd., London

Evans, P. (1975) - Motivation (Essential Psychology). Methuen, London

Handy, C. (1993) - Understanding Organisations. Penguin Books, London

Heckhausen, H. (1967) - The Anatomy of Achievement Motivation. Academic Press, London

Hertzberg, F. (1966) - Work and the Nature of Man. World Publishing, Cleveland, Ohio

Maslow, A.H. (1970) - Motivation and Personality. Harper & Row, New York

Petty, G. (1993) - Teaching Today. Stanley Thornes (Publishers) Ltd., Cheltenham

Rowntree, D. (1987) - Assessing Students: How shall we know them? Kogan Page, London

Vroom, V.H. (1964) - Work and Motivation. Wiley, New York

CHAPTER 4
Setting Objectives

RODNEY PEYTON & LYNNE ALLERY

INTRODUCTION

IN CHAPTER TWO, setting objectives was identified as an essential principal of adult education. These objectives guide learning by giving it both focus and direction. In this chapter, the detail and the practicalities of setting objectives will be discussed in greater depth. Confusion often arises between the terms aim, goal and objective and so these will be explained. The three essential elements in defining objectives will be reviewed in relation to four particular domains of behaviour.

RATIONALE FOR USING OBJECTIVES

Teachers in the professions are now under more pressure than ever before to both fulfil their service commitment *and* provide 'quality' teaching time. Many learners find themselves in a similar situation with a constant battle to find protected time for educational purposes. Combined with this there are financial constraints.

High-tech teaching resources that often help in the teaching process may be out of the question from a financial point of view. Generally, they are not readily portable from one teaching environment to another.

In order to use time and resources (including human ones) in the most efficient manner, it is important to understand a particular teaching episode's purpose or end point. This end point is defined as the objective. From the learner's point of view, this is what the learner will know or be able to do by the end of the session. It is important that the end point be measurable against his or her levels of knowledge and skill prior to the teaching episode. Achievement, or otherwise, of the objective allows student, teacher and institution to evaluate the learning process. In other words, it helps to define the educational input's 'value added' to the learner.

DEFINITIONS

At this stage, it is appropriate to clearly define the three terms objective, goal and aim. An aim is a broad statement of intent. It reflects the ideals and aspirations of a profession, an institution or indeed those who wish to organise a particular course or teaching episode. An example would be 'to generally increase the level of surgical skill in management of breast cancer'.

On the other hand, by setting a goal one defines how this could be achieved. The aim of increasing the level of surgical skill in breast cancer could be realised through the national or regional level development of courses in breast surgery. Alternatively, distance learning courses could be provided including the production of appropriate textbooks. In their expectations of a particular student or branch of the profession, the profession, the examining boards, the institutions, or the general population determines the intended outcomes for such activities. Therefore, in general terms, a goal is the destination of learning. This usually includes some time element.

Objectives can be divided into two broad groups. The first are *specific* objectives. These clearly define what the learner should be able to do by the end of the teaching session relative to what they could not do before. Objectives must be clearly defined from a learner's perspective. Specific objectives are the most useful in the learning process since, once they are clearly stated, they can be fully discussed in advance of a teaching episode by any stakeholder, be they student, teacher, institution or even the public at large,. Thus, misconceptions can then be ironed out and points of contention, including the setting of priorities agreed in advance. Such tightly defined objectives are especially useful in training schemes at the lower levels of the educational process.

Contemporaneous or sequential grouping of such objectives give a clear overview of a course, with the individual objectives being used as signposts in the achievement of the overall aim. This allows the ongoing matching of expectations with performance and any necessary course corrections to be made during the process. If such objectives are not clearly defined then it becomes increasingly difficult to provide indicators of achievement. Further, clearly defined objectives can be prioritised into categories such as 'must know', 'should know', 'could know', or 'would be of interest'. Such prioritisation gives a degree of meaning to the knowledge.

Where clear end points can be achieved and directly assessed, specific objectives are easiest to define with skills. Other learning goals may involve a life-long developmental process. Although, under such circumstances the objectives of individual teaching episodes are not so easy to define they should not be ignored. This is most obvious in discussing social issues such as ethics where there really is no defined 'end point'. Only checking samples of performance in order to give some idea of overall development can really assess progress.

The other main category is teaching or *general* objectives. Based on specific objectives translated to the teacher's point of view these help structure the educational episode, to determine the mode of teaching and establish the form which assessment should take.

DOMAINS

These are defined as the various 'fields' of behaviour. These encompass knowledge, skills, attitude and social behaviour. Before starting the teaching process consideration has to be given to what the learner must actually achieve. In order to make this task efficient it is useful to define the intended learning outcomes as closely as possible into these four fields of behaviour. Each will now be discussed in greater detail.

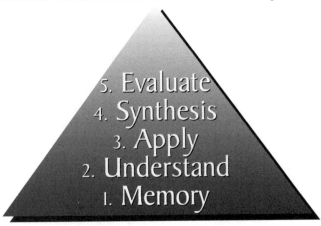

Fig. 1 HIERARCHY OF KNOWLEDGE

Knowledge is a background of facts and interactions between facts that should lead to an understanding of the material being learned. In order to help understanding it needs to be placed in context. This should eventually promote the ability to apply that understanding in different circumstances. At a basic level of factual knowledge it is relatively easy to define clear end points. By the end of the episode the learner either does or does not possess the basic material. For instance, this may be the normal level of haemoglobin or the branches of the facial nerve. Higher levels of knowledge and understanding are required to discuss managing patients with a low haemoglobin or facial paralysis and in evaluating or auditing results.

Such knowledge is not defined easily. It depends on the learner following a logical process and obtaining other pieces of information as indicated. Clearly, it requires 'knowledge in action', facts and experience, combined with judgement. At this level there may be more than one right outcome. In assessing such cases one would look at the development of a logical pathway towards an end point. This is very difficult to define and evidence can only be sampled.

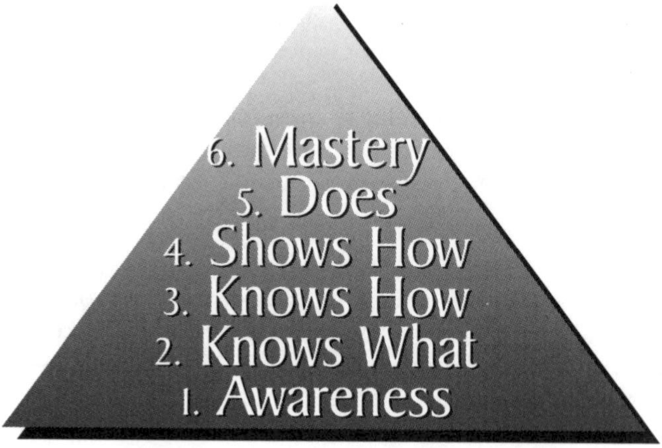

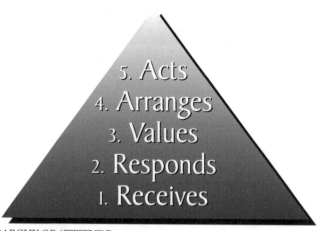

Fig. 2 HIERARCHY OF SKILLS

Objectives in the *skills* domain may be the easiest to set. Generally, they can be written with a view to obtaining 100 per cent mastery. A logical sequence to an end point can be described in terms of the standards and conditions under which the skill should be carried out. Even here, at the highest levels of mastery where learned skills are used to develop other techniques or to deal with abnormal situations the end point of learning cannot be defined except in broad terms. For instance, did the patient survived the procedure without any significant complications? The clinical auditing process attempts to look at this problem by comparing outcomes between individuals within or across units.

Fig. 3 HIERARCHY OF ATTITUDE

Attitude reflects the value placed on the body of knowledge or particular skill. Perhaps, the most difficult field to understand, it may well be the most important. Unless the learning is valued it is likely to be short term in nature. Knowledge levels diminish quickly and actual clinical performance falls far short of any initial competence demonstrated whilst under instruction. Because objectives in this field are so diffi-cult to define in assessment they are often glossed over. This bears out 'McNamara's Fallacy' whereby assessors tend to make what is measurable important, as opposed to making what is important measurable.

Attitude is the linchpin of any profession, forming as it does the basic ethic or accept-ed code of practice. Therefore, it needs a very high priority in any assessment process.

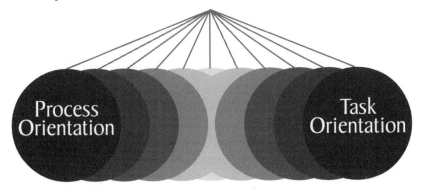

Fig. 4 SOCIAL DOMAIN

The *social* domain reflects the extent of collaboration in a group context. This can be represented by a scale. At one end there is total process orientation with very little drive towards achieving a specific task. At the other end the whole drive is towards achievement of the task at the expense of any attempt at group involvement. Objec-tives in this domain vary with the nature of the task. A life or death decision demands an immediate drive towards task achievement. On the other hand, working in wards with other professionals and patients requires much more attention to the overall process. Due weight must be given to the thoughts and feelings of all participants.

From the teaching and learning process point of view, it becomes obvious that the tight definition of specific objectives is most appropriate at the lowest levels of knowl-edge. Skills and attitude are seen in the early, formative parts of a training process. At a later stage they are all required to interact. It can be difficult to tease apart each ele-ment. Here the terms, 'knowledge', 'skills', 'attitudes' and 'social skills' translate into behaviour types that have the same meaning but reflect the more complex interac-tions.

Therefore, *Cognitive* behaviour is based on knowledge. It implies knowledge in action and at higher levels requires both the knowledge base and an attitude (or ethic) towards the use of that knowledge.

Psychomotor behaviour requires the basic dexterity of the skill correctly performed coupled with the knowledge of how and when to use the skill. (An example of this might be dealing with operating procedure complications.) As well, there should be an ethical attitude towards using the skill. This is reflected in contrasting the three terms - ability, competence and performance. If learners can develop skills they must have had innate ability. Training should imply they have been able to demonstrate competence in a par-ticular technique. However, this does not necessarily reflect unsupervised performance in the real world. This requires not only possessing the skill and knowing how to use it, but that knowledge and skill are properly valued. There must be a strong internal drive to try and overcome other external factors that may influence performance. Otherwise, external factors simply become an excuse for inadequate performance.

Interpersonal behaviour implies the ability to work with others, both contributing to the process and accepting the input of others within the team context. This becomes vital in the higher levels of postgraduate education especially with continuing professional development amongst peer groups. An expert in one field in which he or she may be regarded as the group teacher or facilitator an individual in another context may not be in the lead role but on the receiving end of the teaching/learning process. This requires an attitude of mind which values the knowledge, skills and the input of others. This is behaviour in the affective domain and is the most fundamental of all, underpinning as it does the other three. It is a vital core to continued professional development.

ELEMENTS

There are three main specific objective elements. These encompass performance, conditions, and standards. *Performance* defines exactly what it is that the learner should know or be able to do by the end of the teaching session, that he or she was not able to do before. *Condition* describes the context in which the skill should be carried out, for instance under direct questioning or in a skills laboratory or in a ward given a patient with a particular history. *Standards* constitute what is regarded as satisfactory performance. This requires some form of statement identifying both the standards' setter and assessor.

These three elements are fairly obvious in dealing with skills. It follows that *performance* becomes the assimilated knowledge base along with *conditions*. For example, putting this knowledge in a clinical situation. *Standards* reflect the application of the knowledge to solve a clinical problem. Attitudinal objectives are concerned with the type of behaviour displayed. *Conditions* cover the practical application of this behaviour, for example, showing that the type of behaviour is used and valued in clinical practice. *Standards* are as judged against the profession's role models.

It is important to monitor so-called 'experts' or role models. While, their knowledge may make them good role models in their own particular speciality, it may do so in the field in which they are asked to teach. For instance, an eminent biochemist may not necessarily be the best tutor in clinical biochemistry. He or she may create false expectations as to the 'need to know' for a particular group of learners. Then again, an extremely skilled surgeon who has developed his own particular techniques may not be the most appropriate person to teach basic surgical skills. Similarly, a doctor who performs robustly in court in a medico-legal context may or may not be the most sensitive in breaking bad news to patients or their relatives. An expert should be carefully evaluated for his ability to impart that knowledge in a meaningful way to learners and not only for his appropriate expertise and his or her experience.

OUTCOMES

Unfortunately, the setting of overall aims and goals is often quite woolly with broad, sweeping and all encompassing statements. In this way, they can be made acceptable to students, teachers, or institutions. Each can interpret the aims and goals from their own point of view. Such lack of definition can, and often does, lead to considerable confusion in course content, individual teaching episodes and the learner's own personal study programme. Accordingly, it is equally difficult to assess achievement in the learning process.

This being so, aims and goals in any teaching episode must be translated into specific objectives for the learner. In other words, there should be a clear definition of what the learner must be able to show or do by the end of the process. This indicates that learning has taken place. Once there is a clearly defined end point it is much easier for the learner to move by his or her chosen method towards achieving that end point. This is far better than working around the subject area with little information as to whether the path chosen matched what was expected. Therefore, objectives are used as a method of directing the thinking process and of making the learning more efficient. A simple demonstration of this might be the wish to purchase a second hand freezer. This could be defined as the objective. Most newspapers have classified sections that contain many advertisements for second-hand freezers. Normally, these would not even be noticed, but once the objective is clearly defined then this focus will reveal many opportunities to purchase.

Teaching is the same. Once the objective is clearly defined for learner and teacher, appropriate focussed efforts can be put into planning how to achieve it through the most appropriate available methods.

SETTING OBJECTIVES

The general cycle of objective setting starts with an agreement of what has to be achieved within the context of the overall aims and goals. In advance of the teaching episode, various constraints, including feasibility and fidelity (relationship between the teaching environment and real situations) can be fully discussed by any stakeholder (student, teacher, institution or the public at large). Clarification can be sought and any points of contention including the setting of priorities can be agreed in advance. Such a process helps to define the mode and the speed of teaching, the resources required and the nature of the assessment. The learner's motivation should be assessed and used as an important tool for the whole learning process. When feasible, it is best to start with overall aims and goals and brainstorm the objectives gradually. In this way one narrows them by agreement until it is possible to specify exactly what the learner should be able to do by the end of the episode, teaching period or course.

This can be done with all stakeholders. However, as far as possible, special weight should be given to the learners themselves so that they fully identify with the intended outcomes. If some individuals do not fully accept overall class or group objectives there can be problems with motivation. At the lowest level of knowledge that is at the skills and attitudes level, it is fairly easy to define what must be learned. After all it makes sense to try and get most learners to a professional institution's required standard.

This minimum required level is not negotiable. It must be possible to accurately measure outcomes. Any difference between these and the original objectives should be highlighted and discussed. If necessary, this could lead to modifying objectives for the next occasion.

Objectives are necessary to set the direction of learning and establish assessable outcomes. If these are inconsistent, inputs to courses, even those in progress, can be changed. Objectives become signposts along the road to learning. They lay down what the student must achieve by at the end of the session and lead to disciplined learning that guides the student even when the teacher is not present. They allow for clear, unambiguous feedback and can give rise to a sense of achievement in the student, the teacher and the institution. In courses, it is vital that such feedback is given to those responsible for students' development since it allows corrections to the process whilst the course is in progress. The signposts are essentially formative although each can have its own specific end point. These can be measured, and the more clearly defined each signpost is then the easier the assessment.

The whole process allows the various constraints on outcomes to become obvious. These constraints include equipment, cost, time and personnel as well as the student's learning capacity at any particular moment. The latter is not necessarily a measure of intelligence. It has to include other issues such as tiredness, distractions, and so on.

Objectives also help determine the teaching mode. Teaching methodology runs on a continuum. It starts from purely didactic methods, (basically passive or reception learning), through guided individual response to apprenticeship and finally, to individual study and responsibility. In the latter the teacher becomes a facilitator rather than a direct source of information.

It is important that objectives state what the student is to learn and not what he or she has been exposed to. This states that the teacher delivered the material but is not a test that any learning has taken place. Therefore, when the objective is clear both the teaching method and the instructor's appropriateness can be assessed. This may lead to the use of other professionals in medical education such as nurses, social workers, statisticians, or even the police.

Methods of assessing students will be discussed more fully in the next chapter. However, it should be obvious that assessment depends on the objectives. Knowledge does not equal power. Power is knowledge in action. Therefore it is much better to make an assessment in the context of practice or at least over a period of time. It is easier to assess groups that have been together and with the same teachers over long periods. The teachers are responsible for assessment or have a close liaison with those making the assessment. Correspondingly, it can be difficult making assessments on a short course, especially if different tutors give their own sessions and leave without forming any particular relationship with the group.

If the objectives are kept fairly constant, assessing the students also gives teachers some feedback by helping to evaluate the course and the teaching skills. Assessment of the same cohort of students in different contexts and with different staff members can inform peer review of particular teachers, departments and even institutions. In terms of the latter it is important that there is a commonality of syllabus across a number of institutions so that external exam results can be compared on a level playing field. It also allows a free exchange of ideas between institutions along with research and development and makes the examination system much more meaningful to prospective employers.

DRAWBACKS OF OBJECTIVES

Finally, it must be pointed out that there are some obvious drawbacks to having tightly defined objectives. If overdone, the teaching episodes can become restrictive for both the students and the teacher. This can lead to confrontation rather than partnership. Tightly defined objectives favour superficial learning driven by assessment and not by the desire to understand and learn. Under such circumstances learners feel bound to a particular pattern in a slavish though generally agreed manner. This does not allow for other equally valid learning outcomes that may not be required at the time. Judgements have to be made about whether or not the achievement is acceptable and against what yardstick it should be measured. Further, the student must value and need the objectives if they are to be taken through to real life. Therefore, training objectives mean more than achieving and demonstrating a level of competence. Future performance in the real world must also be taken into account. This requires that the learner values the objectives.

65

CONCLUSION

In this chapter, we discussed the need for organised teaching experiences. At the same time, we acknowledged that not all education is organised. Much of it has no clearly defined end point. This must be taken into account when looking at the higher levels of 'understanding' or 'attitudes'. Here, freedom of expression is necessary. Yet, defining an end point is very difficult since it must be open and allow development to continue. By not allowing for this freedom of expression and thought, very tight objectives trivialise and dehumanise the issues. On the other hand, showing some movement in the desired direction at these higher levels is necessary and the general pathways should be set out. Therefore, there is a continuum between the very tight objectives expected in a lecture or low level training episode and the much looser overall course objectives and very wide open directives of life-long learning.

PUTTING THIS CHAPTER INTO ACTION

Objectives clearly define a pathway and guide both the learner's and teacher's thinking. They must be set within the context of the aims and goals of the academic institution or profession. After this they must be translated into specific learning objectives. The more tightly defined these become the more discussion one needs to urge all stakeholders to agree on them. Those on the receiving end have to be convinced of their validity. This receiving end includes both students and teachers. Lack of motivation in either seriously damages the teaching and learning process. One way of achieving consensus is to brainstorm the particular objectives with representatives of those directly involved.

Once these have been further refined, five specific questions should be used to check the validity of objectives:

1. Do they appear to reflect appropriately all intended outcomes and do they sit well with the present state of knowledge?

2. Are they measurable and are the outcomes clear?

3. Are they attainable by the intended learners and in the time available?

4. Do they reflect the institution and the public's intent?

5. Do they fit with the principles of learning?

This should lead to the formation of general teaching objectives through which the specific learning objectives can be developed.

The next step is to achieve a clear and honest statement of the present position. This requires the learner's trust. They must feel secure that any acknowledged deficit in their knowledge base is used positively rather than negatively. This level of trust depends on the ethos of the institution and the long term history of the learning process.

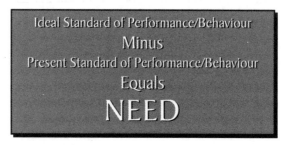

Ideal Standard of Performance/Behaviour

Minus

Present Standard of Performance/Behaviour

Equals

NEED

Fig. 5 SETTING OBJECTIVES

Once the present level of knowledge is understood by all concerned then the gap between this and teaching objectives can be identified. If the gap is regarded as too large it may be narrowed by reducing the level of the particular course's teaching objective or raising the entry level knowledge base. This may also suggest prior preparation of the learner by pre-reading. It may be appropriate preparation for a seminar to say, 'Before we discuss the management of a case of jaundice tomorrow, I will expect you to have read the appropriate chapter in your textbook'. In terms of courses, needs might include prior assessment, such as previous certification, demonstrating an assessed level of professional knowledge, the use of a pre-test or discussion with individuals or groups on the first meeting.

Once the gap has been defined the 'tension' to close it stimulates the learning process. The size of the gap indicates whether one learning objective is sufficient or whether a number of sequential objectives or signposts are needed. These may be developed from the learner's and teacher's past experience, the history of other courses or it may be agreed by the group as before. They are turned into specific statements of objectives which can be prioritised into groups such as 'must know', 'should know', 'could know' and 'nice to know'. There should now be a clear set of learners' objectives prioritised for a course, that may take several days to develop, or a one hour teaching session that can be sorted out in a matter of minutes. It is only after the objectives have been listed that the appropriate methods of teaching and assessment can be worked out.

SUGGESTED FURTHER READING

Beard, R. & Hartley, J. (1984) – Teaching & Learning in Higher Education. PCP Limited, London

Gronlund, N.E. & Linn, R.L. (1990) – Measurement & Evaluation in Teaching. MacMillan Publishing Company, New York

Ramsden, P. (1992) – Learning to Teach in Higher Education. Routledge, London

Rowntree, D. (1981) – Developing Courses for Students. PCP Limited, London

TenBrink, T.D. (1986) – Writing Instructional Objectives. Cooper J. (editor). Classroom Teaching Skills 3rd Edition. D.C. Heath Lexington, Mass.

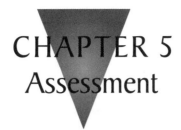

CHAPTER 5
Assessment

DUNCAN HARRIS

INTRODUCTION

IN UNITED KINGDOM practice, assessment refers to the process of checking an individual's progress and attainment. A vital part of any teaching role, assessment may also provide a means of measuring the teacher's performance a as well.

This chapter looks at assessment and asks three fundamental questions: Why?, For whom?, and By what means? It then looks in more detail at various assessment methods such as multiple choice questions or Objective Structured Clinical Examinations (OSCE). It concludes with a set of guidelines for producing an assessment.

THE NATURE OF ASSESSMENT

Most readers will have taken higher level university entry examinations as well as a driving test. Let us look at these two assessments in a little more detail.

The higher examinations are there to assess knowledge and ability to apply that knowledge at the end of a course. However, the examination has another purpose. For instance, who uses the results and how? Key users are higher education institutions with a limited number of places. They use the grades to select their students for the next year. The institutions use the results to compare candidates.

The driving test is different. There are a series of smaller parts, each of which must be achieved (for example, highway code test, three point turn, reversing, emergency stop). The tester looks for a fixed level of performance on each part of the test, in other words, there are criteria laid down that must be met. It is possible for an examiner to pass every candidate.

As well, the key users for these assessments are different. Let us consider the higher examinations first. We have already identified one audience, the higher education institution. Other key users are the candidates themselves. The school or college where they learned is another key user. If the results are good for all candidates, this will be used for publicity in order to try to get more learners to choose that school or college. Other key users could include parents, and school or college finance providers as well as its governors who use it as a means of monitoring teaching. It is difficult to see who has the ownership of these assessments and results, as clearly there are a large number of stakeholders.

The driving test is really providing a licence to drive on the roads and obviously the general public have an important stake in the process. Candidates and driving schools (again for publicity and for monitoring of teaching) will use the results. The ownership is clearly the government on behalf of the public.

The timing of the assessment is also interesting in each of these cases. The driving test occurs at the end of the instruction. The assessment of much higher education occurs during the course (course work, projects) and at the end of the course. In this way, the assessment monitors both the process and its end. Timing depends on assessment requirements.

Some assessments help learners. Teachers and tutors mark and comment on assignments to help learning. It is not to provide a label for further progress or a licence to perform.

Clearly, the assessment's purpose needs to be considered before it is designed.

WHY ASSESS?

The two assessments that were referred to in the previous section label the candidate with a pass or a grade. Often called *summative assessments*, they are intended to identify what has been learned at a particular time and not predict future performance. The evidence is that entry level university results do not correlate well with degree results, even in the same subject. They are not designed to predict performance. The Driving Test does not predict future performance as a driver and prediction would require a different sort of assessment that was designed specifically for that purpose. In the early days of computers it was realised that logical thinking was a crucial requirement for programmers and so logical thinking tests were devised to predict future performance. The computer industry still uses tests that predict performance when selecting future employees.

Before publication, results from higher education examinations are fed into a computer to generate a set of data that relates to a normal distribution which gives a bell shaped curve. The distribution of the results is thus scaled to a normal distribution and such assessments are called *norm-referenced*. Assessments are designed specifically to produce that distribution.

The driving test is different. The tester looks for a fixed level of performance based on the criteria specified. Such assessments are called *criterion-referenced* with the assessments designed so that the criteria are met.

The other type of assessment briefly mentioned in the previous section was the sort that a teacher or tutor sets a learner in order to give an opportunity for comments on progress. This can be very easily referenced against a population or set criteria, or referenced against the learner's previous performance which is termed self-referencing. An assessment designed to help progress is called formative assessment. Such assessments can be formal, for example an essay or a set of calculations, or informal such as questions asked in the classroom. Not only do these tests give the learner feedback, they inform the teacher on difficulties widespread within a group.

Clearly, there are important decisions to be made about assessment before they are designed:

- Are they only to be at the end or also during the learning process?
- Are they to be norm, criterion, or self-referenced?
- For whom are the results intended as the main audience?
- Are the assessments for the benefit of learners to help their learning or are they just a means of labelling a learner?

FOR WHOM?

We have already looked at some of the possible assessment stakeholders. Whether the assessment is for a two-day course or a five-year course, there will be a variety of them.

The two-day course is financed usually by an organisation (such as a Hospital Trust). If the Trust finds that people are more successful when they are sent to a course at place A rather than at place B, they are likely to send their future attendees to the former course. The assessment is used to evaluate the course's effectiveness.

Similarly, when learners have a choice, they often consult colleagues about the choice of venue. There may be other factors that are now considered such as food, accommodation, kindliness and helpfulness of course staff. Again, these are being used for evaluation. However, if the record of the centre is that a large number fails, then these other factors will pale into insignificance.

Certain assessments give the right to practise and have much more impact on the general public. These are more likely to be carefully monitored by a controlling body and updated as new techniques are introduced into common practice.

Peers will also be interested in one another's progress. Not only does this confer credibility (or otherwise) on the assessment, it also provides information about the expectations.

One past problem was that assessments were kept secret and control lay almost exclusively with the examiner. Candidates did not know what was expected. Public scrutiny of assessments and the financial implications of successive failures caused the system to be questioned with the result that assessments became more open and the rules of the game made clearer.

Therefore, assessment design needs to take into account the stakeholders. In addition, the assessment format must be considered early in the design process.

BY WHAT MEANS?

In spite of the wide array of assessment methods (these will be introduced in the next section), there are only three means, written, oral and observation, that can be used for assessment:

—*Written* assessment can cover a wide range from ticks in boxes, through one word answers, to essays and even theses. A key consideration in professional assessments is how near the assessment is to reality. This is one aspect of validity. Validity means asking whether the assessment measures what it set out to. Height can be used as a measure of weight, but clearly it is open to many errors.

—*Oral* assessments have been used for hundreds of years but these depend on the assessor. The evidence is that there is considerable inconsistency between examiners, and this makes for poor reproducibility. Reproducibility relates to the consistency between examiners and the results achieved by examinees undertaking the same examination at different times.

—Like the driving test, many professional assessments require the demonstration of *observation* skills. Sometimes video recordings enhance observation by allowing replay of the performance and analysis of the skill. However, this obviously takes longer and requires a ratio of, at least, one examiner per candidate. The resources may become too stretched to carry out much assessing, so the feasibility and manageability must be considered too.

Combinations of written, oral and observation will be further discussed next.

Written

Written assessments are particularly useful for assessing cognitive learning. Also, while useful for some aspects of affective learning, they are of limited use when assessing psychomotor or inter-personal aspects.

Three simple types of assessment will be considered. These are multiple-choice questions (MCQ), multiple short answer questions (MSA) and essay questions with many variations on each.

MCQ

Three approaches will be outlined briefly. These use four or five options, multiple true false, extended matching. The four or five options item is common in the USA. An example follows:

Plants are categorised according to their life cycle. In the UK, the petunia would be treated as a:
a) Annual ....❏
b) Biennial ....❏
c) Biannual ....❏
d) Perennial ....❏

72

The options have been presented in order of word length. Other alternatives would be putting the shortest first, or using alphabetical order. The obvious basis removes the idea that there is a trick in the question.

This type of question is best designed by asking learners an open question. Using the answers that they have given, the key (correct answer) and the distracters can be selected.

When using a sequence of questions, it is important to ensure that the key is not always in the same location (say, option C).

A variety of marking approaches is used. For example, one mark for the correct option, zero marks for any others. Alternatively, 2-4 marks for the best answer, 1 for possible answers, 0, or even a negative number for an obviously incorrect answer.

The evidence suggests that whatever system is used the rank order of candidates hardly changes. The single mark for the correct answer is the easiest to manage.

A multiple true false approach would be as follows:

> *Plants are categorised according to their life cycle. In the UK, the following would be the appropriate life cycle:*
>
> *a) Aster..............................biannual.....................................* ❏ True ❏ False
> *b) Mysembrianthemum.......annual...* ❏ True ❏ False
> *c) Petunia............................perennial...................................* ❏ True ❏ False
> *d) Polyanthus......................annual...* ❏ True ❏ False
> *e) Rose................................biennial.....................................* ❏ True ❏ False
> *f) Wallflower.......................perennial...................................* ❏ True ❏ False

Each item would be marked true or false. Marks are usually allocated as one per statement with a deduction of three to allow for guessing (in other words you should get three correct by guessing!)

An extended matching type would be like:

> **THEME: GROWING PLANTS.**
>
> *Options:*
>
> | | |
> |---|---|
> | a) Acid soil | i) High calcium content |
> | b) Alkaline soil | j) High potassium content |
> | c) Good humus content | k) Lack of trace elements |
> | d) Good nitrogen content | l) Full sun |
> | e) Dry conditions | m) Full shade |
> | f) Moist conditions | n) Sun or shade |
> | g) Wet conditions | o) Need regular feeding |
> | h) Water logged conditions | p) Need little or no feeding |

Plants have different growing patterns and environmental needs. For each plant, select the appropriate growing requirements and environmental needs. Each option may be used once, more than once or not at all.

- Cabbages are seen to have yellowing leaves and with hearts lacking body. Identify the causes of this poor growth.
- Hellebores require certain conditions to ensure the best possible growth. Identify those conditions.

With variations within a species, it may be better to give the specific names of varieties. This type of question has potential in medical situations. It can be used as a problem-solving question where a patient and the type of drug to be used are identified in the options.

The general advantage of MCQ is that they can be designed for marking either by a non-expert using a template or they can be designed for use with an Optical Mark Reader. Since both cases are easy to administer, easy to mark and make providing the scores easy there is little chance of marking errors.

The disadvantages are that they are difficult to design, more difficult to use for higher levels of learning, there are clues to the correct answer; and they sometimes can be far removed from reality.

SOME GUIDELINES FOR SETTING MCQ FOLLOW:

1. If the stem is in the form of an incomplete sentence, each choice must complete the sentence using correct grammar.
2. Avoid negative stems since they may lead to double negatives and are unnecessarily difficult to interpret; testing whether something is not so, does not demonstrate whether the student knows what actually is! However the ruling out of a diagnosis would obviously be a sensible in a medical context.
3. Avoid statements open to more than one interpretation.
4. All common phrases should be in the stem.
5. If giving four or five options, the stem should contain a verb. Constructed in such a way that the correct response is immediately suggested from the stem, thus reference to the choices is mere confirmation.
6. Be careful that the use of singulars or plurals in the stem does not lead to correct answers by linking the stem to, say, a singular choice while the distracters are plural.
7. Try to set choices that are all plausible. The distracters should be logical and in most cases based on known errors.
8. Make sure that all choices are plausible in construction.
9. Keep all choices as short as possible to reduce reading. The style should be simple and direct. Where extended matching items are used, practise should be provided with the type of item.
10. Where there is only one correct option make sure that only one statement is correct and clearly the best choice.
11. If there is a logical order to the choices arrange them in that order (for example, alphabetical, order of magnitude, length of statement).
12. Avoid technical terms in the distracters that are unlikely to be known to the candidates. Never introduce nonsense words or terms.
13. Avoid grouping choices in opposite pairs.
14. Avoid overlapping choices.
15. Avoid synonymous distracters.
16. The choice of 'none of the above' is sometimes used, but it should generally be avoided. It should not be used as the correct answer.

74

MSA

Short answer questions need a word or a short phrase as an answer. For example:

List the four types of growing cycle for plants:

1 _____   2 _____

3 _____   4 _____

It is possible to state a scenario and ask several short answer questions for the one case. Such questions are multiple short answer questions.

There must be a marking scheme for this type of question.

- The advantage of this type of question is that there is potential for making a beginning in the addressing of the higher levels of learning. In addition, it is more realistic and learners have to identify the answers themselves.
- The disadvantages are that learners may not understand what is required, and markers may, not only have different views on acceptable answers, they may be inconsistent from one script to the next.

There will be a delay before any results are known. It is important that either each script is double marked or that there be some other system of monitoring examiners to reduce errors.

There can be extended matching items, for example, where there is a diagram needing to be labelled or a table/matrix with blank spaces to be completed.

HERE ARE SOME GUIDELINES FOR SETTING SHORT ANSWER QUESTIONS:

1. Ask only for important relevant information, not non-essentials.
2. Make the sentence structure as simple as possible so that the question is clear to all candidates.
3. State and qualify the question unmistakably so that a single response is correct.
4. Limit the space allocation for each answer to encourage a single word or short phrase.
5. Make sure that all answers have equal or stated weighting.
6. Provide a prepared answer sheet for all candidates to use. Construct it so that it is easy for examiners to mark.
7. For incomplete statements do not over-mutilate sentences by leaving too many blanks.
8. For incomplete statements do not choose omitted words that are interdependent.
9. For an extended matching item limit the number of items in one column to six or so.
10. For an extended matching item clarify the theme clear, the options, the statement and the decisions to be made.

ESSAY

These are probably familiar to most readers. They vary from a structured question (for example, with a definition, a description, a calculation, and a short sting in the tail) to a single question such as: 'Discuss the merits and demerits of installing mains drainage into a village.'

The advantage of this type of question is that it has potential for scanning all the levels of learning in the cognitive domain. It is also nearer to reality. In effect, it is more valid. It may be easier sitting all the candidates down at once and getting the assessment over in one, two or three hours.

The disadvantages are that even with an agreed mark scheme, it is likely that different markers will allocate different marks. Thus, there are problems of inter-marker reliability and marking time is increased considerably. There is more need to check the marking and the additions carried out by markers. Final marks are delayed and managing the marking and the collating of data is not easy.

The other essay question takes the form of an extended report, such as a project report. The report is completed over a period of time. It may include a log or diary of events or it may be just a report at the end. The same problems arise as for essays, except that reality is increased. Marking becomes even more difficult.

SOME GUIDELINES FOR ESSAY TYPE QUESTIONS FOLLOW:

1. State clearly whether accurate answers or estimates (or precise figures or sketches) are required.
2. Avoid questions that can be answered by a single word or a short phrase.
3. Use the words: 'discuss', 'explain', 'compare' only when deliberately aiming a the higher levels of the cognitive domain (for example as the last part of a structured question or as a stand alone question).
4. Avoid negative questions and statements. They lead to double negatives in the answer and these are difficult to interpret.
5. Use short sentences.
6. Avoid ambiguity.
7. Avoid technical terms that are unfamiliar to the candidates.
8. Display any data clearly and together.
9. For calculations state the requirements, for example: 'state any formulae used and present initial substitutions'.
10. Ensure that a structured question develops through the cognitive levels from lower to higher levels.
11. Do not ask questions where the candidates have to spend a lot of time on trivia.
12. Compose a detailed model answer. Identify important statements, steps or parts of graphs/diagrams by underlining or circling them. Marks should be allocated for each part and detailed within that part.
13. Marks given for each section should be shown in the question paper.
14. State the anticipated answering time for the question taking into account that candidates will be writing the answer under examination conditions, or identfy the time expected to be spent if the essay is to be done in their own time.

76

15. Ensure that the expectations and time required are the same as others in the same assessment.

Examiners can be trained to carry out all these types of questions. For MCQ, the training would focus on the setting of questions. For the other types of assessment, the focus would be on marking sample scripts.

Oral

Most will be familiar with oral examinations or viva voces. This type of assessment is often used in association with another form such as a project report, a dissertation, or a thesis. Orals are probably open to more abuses, less validity and lower reliability than any other from of assessment. The validity can be low because the questions do not relate to the learner's experience. For example, there may be questions about an obscure operation that the candidate is unlikely to have seen or heard about. The reliability can be low because there is no agreed marking procedure between different examiners. It weighs heavily on examiners and candidates' time so it is also unwieldy. One potential for orals is to assess attitudes, that is the affective domain. This is a specialised approach needing reference to a specialised text.

Orals can be of two types, structured or unstructured. Structured orals have an agenda of questions planned before the oral takes place. The questions focus on particular levels of learning. Some examples would be:

*State, name, list*_____these suggest a recall from memory.

*Compare, how are these common?*_____these suggest some inference, so are at the comprehension level.

*How can you use it? How could you*_____?suggesting necessity to apply or to analyse.

*Can you think of a new approach to*_____? *What do you suggest if*_____? a higher level still where there is synthesis.

*Will this work? Is there a better solution?*_____these go a bit further and require evaluation too.

Structured orals must clearly identify the level for which questions will be designed. This needs careful preparation and it can be useful to have on hand lower level subsidiary questions if the candidate cannot answer those at a higher level. Subsequent questions should try to attain the higher level again.

A checklist of questions and the expected outcomes are useful. The marks allocated, the priorities (or weightings) of parts of the questions and the means of deducing a final mark or grade must be designed *before* questions are used in an oral. Video recordings of student responses are useful for training examiners.

Unstructured orals use the candidate's responses to elicit the next questions. Clearly, there are problems if this type of assessment is to be used as a major part of the allocation of marks towards, say, a degree. The unstructured orals tend to be used for idiosyncratic follow-up assessments. These may be after the individual's project or a major piece of practical work. In such instances, that assessment may enhance learning rather than allocate grades or marks. The examiner analyses the learner's performance (perhaps using a video recording of it). Questions can be asked that may be specific to technique, to theoretical background or to taking the learner on to more advanced and complex approaches.

GUIDELINES FOR ORALS:

1. State the assessment's purpose.
2. Clearly state candidate's expectations.
3. Where the assessment is based on a previous activity, it should usefully enhance candidate's learning.
4. Do not use assessments that require candidates to spend a lot of time on trivia.
5. The assessment should bring together previous learning and extend expeience.
6. Compose a clear framework for the assessment (perhaps using a matrix).
7. State how the assessment will be carried out (for example one tutor using a checklist).
8. Compose a schedule or checklist, relating this to the framework.
9. Ensure that a clear simple statement of the assessment procedures is available to the examiners and to the candidates.
10. Ensure that examiners know how the marks will be allocated from the checklist, schedule, or framework.
11. Ensure that questions used are unambiguous and focus on one idea at a time.
12. Ensure that questions are simple and brief.
13. Ensure that candidates can admit to not knowing an answer without loss of face. Marking could reflect this. For example, a spontaneous answer would receive x marks. An answer following slight prompting - y marks. With heavy prompting - z marks. This is especially useful in items that are heavily weighted.
14. Ensure that words and phrases in a question do not influence (lead) the answer.
15. Avoid negative questions. The ruling out of a diagnosis could be an exception.
16. Organise the order and sequence of questions, including probes.
17. Ensure that the procedures, schedules, framework are checked by other tutors and examiners before use.
18. Try out the questions on surrogate candidates.
19. Ensure that the layout of the environment is stipulated so that it is not too threatening to candidates.

Observation

Observation is the only technique available for most practical activities. It can be used for teamwork. As for orals, the approach can be structured or unstructured. The former is more suitable for grading and marking, although it is also useful for learning purposes. The unstructured approach is only suitable for enhancing learning. Again, the task to be assessed must be analysed carefully. For example, a simple set of design rules would be as follows:

DEFINING WHAT IS TO BE TESTED:
- Identify the problems the student should be able to deal with or resolve.
- For each problem, define the clinical tasks in which the student is expected to be competent.
- Prepare a matrix to guide the selection of problems and tasks to be included in the assessment procedure.

79

SELECTION OF ASSESSMENT METHOD(S)
- Aim for a method that most closely represents reality and is appropriate for the task being assessed.
- The clinical task should dictate the assessment method that is to be used.
- Recognise that there are constraints to selecting the best assessment methods.
- Other issues to be considered include, checklists and rating scales, scoring procedures (pass/fail, score per case), observation and recording procedures, weighting, combining scores, bias, trivialising, and reporting scores.
- A matrix can ensure that the candidate does not have many assessments on history-taking and, for example, no assessments on treatment and team relationships. The matrix can be a basis for the observation approaches to be used to ensure that there is adequate coverage of all aspects without undue duplication. It may also be used with advantage during oral assessments (Figure 1).

	History	Physical examination	Tests and procedures	Diagnostic acumen	Treatment	Judgement & skill for care including continuing care	Responsibilities as practitioner	Team relationships	Relationships with patients
Gynaecology									
Obstetrics									
Paediatrics									
Terminal illness									
Trauma									
Cardio-vascular									
Orthopaedics									
Neurology									
Etc.									

Fig. 1 TYPICAL MATRIX FOR UNDERGRADUATE ASSESSMENT

A clinical assessment for teaching purposes could look like this:

> PROBLEM SOLVING (Acute Myocardial Infarction)
> *(This is a teaching [formative] assessment for which there can be up to 30 min.)*
> *Expectations*
> 1. Perform a rapid evaluation of the patient with possible AMI, including ABC assessment of clinical status, physical examination and history, vital signs and a 12-lead ECG.
> 2. Know the major indications and the exclusion criteria for thrombolytic therapy.
> 3. Know the ECG criteria for AMI that merit the use of thrombolytic therapy.
> 4. Know the major actions, indications, and contra-indications for medications for the AMI Logarithm.
> 5. Recognise and properly treat the listed arrhythmic complications of AMI.
> *Unacceptable actions*
> 1. Failure to consider and properly evaluate (ECG, monitor, history, and physical examination) a patient with acute chest pain suggestive of AMI. Failure to obtain a 12-lead ECG early for patients with possible AMI. Failure to initiate oxygen and other indicated medicines for patient with AMI. Failure to recognise exclusion criteria for the use of thrombolytic therapy.
> 2. Administration of contra-indicated medications.
> *Resources*
> • Active mannequin with tutor to provide data as student requests.
> • Detailed equipment listed in course manual.

It is important to note that there is a clear identification of the resources required as well as the expectations from the assessment. The actual checklist for such an assessment might look like:

Critical Action	Completed	Not completed	Comments
Rapidly assesses ABCs			
Rapidly determines clinical status with physical examination, history and vital signs.			
Immediately orders 12-lead ECG			
Applies indications and exclusion criteria for use of thrombolytics.			
Applies ECG criteria for AMI to patient.			
Consider other interventions and medications.			
Treats complications of AMI, including most common arrhythmia.			

Fig. 2 ASSESSMENT CHECKLIST

The assessment does not allocate marks but is used as a means of helping the learner enhance performance. A similar grid can be used to allocate marks. There would have to be certain decisions such as the following.

- Which actions are essential?
- Which actions are more important (worth twice the mark allocation)?
- What marks will be allocated, if any, if the sequence is wrong?
- What marks will be allocated if prompting is required?
- Are any marks to be allocated for confidence and overall performance rather than to each element?

Until decisions are made on these aspects, it is difficult for two examiners to come up with similar grades for the same performance by the same candidate.

Examiner training is crucial to ensure consistency between examiners and to improve reliability. Designed checklists and marking procedures are used with video recordings to improve performance.

COMBINATIONS OF APPROACHES

OBJECTIVE STRUCTURED CLINICAL EXAMINATION (OSCE)

The Objective Structured Clinical Examination or circuit test is organised so that candidates spend 5 to 10 minutes at each of 15 to 20 stations. It is intended to measure specific elements of learning at each station. The OSCE is a framework or template for the administration of a number of different methods. Generally, it is agreed that it is best used to assess practical, observable skills and abilities.

In other words, it is not best used for things that can be done more efficiently in other ways such as, for example, using one station to deliver computer-based MCQs that are answered on screen is probably not an efficient use of the OSCE format. Checking the ability to carry out a simple technique would be a better use. The station should have the required equipment, mannequin, or stimulator and the candidate is observed carrying out the procedure by an examiner with a checklist.

Further stations may include more observation of skills or problems that need to be solved perhaps with a video introduction followed by 'What do you do next?' Here, the examiner may use an interactive but structured oral assessment with a checklist. The OSCE approach relates particularly to criterion-referenced assessment wherein expectations for the design of each station are clearly stated. The matrix approach introduced earlier in the chapter is particularly useful for the design of this type of assessment.

OSCEs can now be electronically scored, just like multiple choice questions. This can be very helpful for large scale OSCEs with many candidates and also allows detailed itemised analysis of cohorts' performance on each station. Then too, this is useful for course feedback for organisers and candidates alike. For example, in one OSCE it was found that the disposal of sharps was a ubiquitous problem and this information was relayed to candidates and teachers alike. However, for groups of 30 or less, electronic scoring is redundant.

Guidelines for OSCE

1. The time available should be decided as well as each station's division of time.
2. The overall purpose of the OSCE should be decided.
3. The purpose of each individual station should be determined (for example: assessment of skill; assessment of diagnostic ability).
4. Each station's needs (for example: space, equipment, seating, examiner(s), individual, or group of learners).
5. The location for the OSCE should take into account the needs for space based on the types of equipment and number of learners.
6. The timing and scheduling of learners between stations.
7. Examiners, learners, and administrators should be briefed.
8. Responsibilities for administrators, technicians, and examiners should be allocated.
9. Identification of means of collecting and collating assessment data.
10. Identify detailed assessment procedures. For example, checklists, interview questions and prompts, for each station.
11. Check all assessment procedures with examiners and trials, with learners' peers.

PROJECTS

The general heading covers any activity where an individual or group is required to carry out an investigation, a problem solving exercise, or a design-and-make type of exercise. The project may be assessed many ways. Some are assessed using only the final report. In other cases, there is a contract between learners and tutors. The assessment relates to the contract and may include observation, either written or oral intermediate reports, self assessments, written report and orals. Again, the project's purpose must be clearly identified. When projects are used towards norm-referenced assessments, they can skew results towards the higher end.

Guidelines for Projects

1. Set learners an assignment that will be useful in their future employment.
2. State the assignment's purpose.
3. State any written report's expected sections.
4. State the expected length (number of words or number of pages of any required report.
5. Do not set an assignment where learners have to spend a long time on non-essentials.
6. Set an assignment that brings together or extends previous learning.
7. State clearly the expectations for learners (for example where intermediate presentations or data are required). The learning contract must be designed.
8. Compose an assessment schedule using levels of learning or other expectations, for example, the learning contract, as a basis.
9. State how the means of assessment will be conducted (for example with the tutor using a schedule and observing during the project report read by supervisor and another tutor.)

10. Compose any detailed checklists that are necessary, relating these to the appropriate framework.
11. Ensure that a clear simple statement of assessment criteria and procedures is available to all tutors involved and to learners.
12. Compose a detailed marking procedure and state performance criteria.
13. Check that time available to learners to carry out the assignment is realistic.
14. Ensure that the assignment, with its mark scheme assesses individual learners to a pre-determined standard.

LOGS AND DIARIES

Although particularly useful for assessments aimed at learning, they can also be used for other assessments. It is a way for a supervisor to decide on comments or grade activities as they are performed. The log, or diary, provides a good basis for discussing a learner's progress and for specifying the activities that they have and have not done. Usually, it is used in association with an oral examination, using the log or diary to identify a basis for discussion.

Guidelines for Logs and Diaries

1. Identify the purpose of the log or diary.
2. Identify of the form of the log or diary.
3. Identify the duration of the use of the log or diary.
4. Identify the follow up to the log or diary (for example, a viva voce on operations (described in the log).
5. Verify the checking during completion by tutors.
6. Identify the expectations from learners.
7. Identify any marking or grading schedule for the log or diary.

PRESENTATIONS

This approach is difficult to use for assessments that provide qualifications. Also, it is useful for assessing team work. An extended team project may require the team to present their results. The presentation may have a general introduction, details, and a conclusion and should be presented in an identified order. The speaker sequence is drawn out of a hat at the presentation. The idea is that each speaker should be able to give any part of the presentation. The presentation should be even, for example there should not be a highly mathematical part that is understood by one participant only.

SIMULATIONS AND GAMES

Using simulations is often appropriate where there is danger in using the real thing. For example, take dangerous chemicals, potential danger to patients or risk to very expensive equipment. For expensive or dangerous activities, simulation may be computer-based. Patient simulations may use a mannequin, a simulator or another person. Sometimes a candidate can do the stimulation required, but has to stop short of some activities such as taking blood or performing a complete abdominal examination including a PR. In such simulations, a combination of methods can be used. Then again, some actions can be described but not performed.

In the USA, human simulation has been developed extensively. Through various tricks and techniques, it is possible to simulate, with high fidelity, a variety of clinical syndromes. Examples include meningitis, abnormal heart rhythms, and unilateral breathing and tremors. Also, patient instructors have been used to give learners detailed feedback on examination techniques. This has worked particularly well for musculo-skeletal and neurological systems.

Simulator use could be part of an OSCE or the ultimate course assessment checking whether learners can carry out cognitive and psychomotor activities to a high level, work as a member of a team and have the right attitude. Again, the assessment's purpose and the method for using simulator checklists and readings must be clearly defined beforehand.

Similar to simulations, games usually involve an element of competition. The most sophisticated games tend to be business games using extensive computer resources. Usually, teams are set up to run competing or different businesses. Other factors can be fed in, some predictable, while others will be subject to chance. Again, these can be used as a basis for assessment. Game expectations and rules are defined clearly, as is the way in which it will be used for assessment purposes.

In spite of the approach to realism, the reproducibility of the group of assessments under the heading *combinations* is usually low. However, reasons for this do not seem to be related to the testing methods as such. Research shows them to be caused by the specificity of clinical competence. Being good at a cardiological examination does not confer much information about a candidate's ability at examining the abdomen. When such techniques are put in the context of real cases there is even less agreement between performance in the two domains. This is the reason why in OSCE a large number of areas of competence must be sampled. Hence, there must be careful consideration of staffing implications since most are heavy on assessors. Also, the OSCE requires a good manager to set up the system and ensure the proper briefing of all examiners and candidates. As well, it is necessary to ensure that all the support staff is present, to have a means of collecting and collating assessment data as it comes in, and to manage assessors and candidates on the appropriate day.

BY WHOM?

Traditionally, teachers or professionals from the same profession as those being trained carry out assessments. Teacher assessment is potentially biased since they may have pre-conceived ideas about individuals' performance during training and learning. The outsider is perceived as not having that bias, but instead may have an immediate reaction to the candidate that colours the assessment. The use of self and peer assessment is less common. The evidence is that self and peer assessment is often more critical than that carried out by teachers and outsiders.

No matter who is used for the procedure, it cannot be emphasised too much that all should be quite clear about:
- The purpose of the assessment.
- The means by which it will be carried out.
- The procedure for decision making.

Where there is more than one examiner for a particular assessment it is normal to have a set marking procedure. The use of moderation procedures is common. The examiners meet before the examination, and are given either simulated or real example assessments marked by all the examiners. Afterwards, the discussion looks at the discrepancies in order to modify and reduce discrepancies. The intention is to improve inter-marker reliability.

Where there is an awarding body for an assessment providing, say a degree or diploma, usually there is, at least, one external examiner whose job it is to carry out further moderation to ensure standards with comparable organisations or institutions are the same each year. The external examiner will be involved from the initial setting of the assessments right through to the final decisions.

New examiners should be trained before they are used. This may involve the setting of multiple choice questions. For other assessments, the use of simulations or scripts with a mark scheme or checklist can be useful for the learning procedures to be used and to emphasise the importance of inter-marker reproducibility.

WHEN?

The assessment's purpose helps determine when it should be set. There is a tendency towards modular courses with assessments during or at the end of each module. One issue to be considered when using modular courses is whether there should be an overall or bridging assessment? Some courses use a module for that purpose, while others use a project type of module or modules that enable the overall assessment to bridge a range of modules.

Course assessments can be used for learning purposes. These are assignments that include practical work, problems, and literature surveys. Their main purpose is to serve as a means of both tutor and learner identifying learning problems. Although, they are often used for that purpose, the same assessments are unsuitable for awarding overall grades and marks. Confusing the purpose neither enhances the learning nor enables a fair grading. The alternative is to identify specific assignments that will be graded or marked. For example, while brief reports of practical work may be required each week, formally written reports at regular intervals are necessary for grading or marks. That assignment may focus on considering the potential errors and difficulties inherent in deducing a clear conclusion. Another report may focus on data presentation.

If all assessments are at the module's end, in a full time course a logjam can cause learners and examiners problems. Often there is only one week between modules yet continuation may depend on success in a previous module. Such a time scale may well be too short to enable marking, moderating and external examining. Some, such as practically oriented modules, may lend themselves to assessment during, rather than at the end, of the module. A module requiring gradual cognitive learning growth and knowledge application or its use for analysis may need to have the assessment near the end.

EXPECTED AND UNEXPECTED OUTCOMES

Assessment can be perceived as a game, that like any other, has explicit rules. The evidence of past assessments enables learners to see how the process will change their behaviour. So, for example, if the assessment is by way of unseen examinations requiring a great deal of rote learning, any attempt during the course to get them to look at applications or come up with diagnosis ideas and solutions will be of only partial interest. Similarly, for a course requiring only a project assessed by a report, there is little point in encouraging the learners to learn facts off by heart.

Evidence suggests that where the tutor sets assessments, learners tend to play a further game. Some learners are able to detect that the tutor has particular interests and ideas that are paramount. These so-called 'cue-seekers' focus their learning in that direction too. Others, the 'cue-deaf' remain blissfully unaware. Generally, cue-seekers perform better, particularly in unseen examinations.

The use of modules also causes the learner to focus on the particular rather than trying to gain any overall or developmental learning. Outcomes are determined by the purposes of those assessments. The clearer the rules of the game are to learners and examiners, the more likely that the learning will produce expected outcomes.

SUMMARY

Assessments are used to inform either the learner or others about the learner's performance. The audiences for an assessment are the first component to be considered. The information the audiences require may be different. Employers may want to know what skills and abilities a potential employee has. They require a detailed, but not too extensive, summary of these attributes. Learners may wish to know what else they need to learn – this is almost the opposite of the information required by the employer. Both may also want to know how the learner performed compared with other learners on that course and also elsewhere. Clearly, there is a conflict between the criterion-referenced and the norm-referenced approaches. Compromises may be needed, or different assessments used for different purposes.

All assessments are based on three approaches. The written or spoken word and observation. The written word varies from MCQ through essay questions to logs, diaries and reports. The assignments may be to enhance learning or to give an element towards a grade or mark. For practical work, observation and the effects of the practical work (a sort of audit) can be used. Oral assessment is useful for exploring ideas in detail or for getting some information about attitudes.

Examiners must have a clear idea about the requirements and the details of the assessment procedure. This is particularly true if there are several examiners examining the same attributes. Training examiners helps to improve the reliability of the assessments. The use of moderation procedures and external examiners can also assist.

It is important to remember that adult learners prefer active involvement. This means using activities relating to experience. For example, these might be case-based approaches. Thus, they reflect on meaningful experiences, clear goals and feedback. These preferences also apply to assessments.

The technical problems associated with assessments are:
- Reliability
- Validity
- Feasibility or manageability.

PUTTING THIS CHAPTER INTO ACTION

All assessments try to simulate a real experience. The nearer the assessment is to reality, the more valid it will be. However, as has been indicated in the previous sections, the more reality there is, the more examiners are needed and the more potential there is for discrepancy between them. Using checklists is a means of reducing this discrepancy and helping to improve reliability. The second problem is reality is heavy on resources such as examiners, equipment, space, and time and thus threatens to make the whole assessment unmanageable. However, the key to all assessments is the examiner and the supporting system.

A set of guidelines can be helpful to enable consistency. For example, when setting up practical exams consider the following:

PROCEDURAL

- Ensure that a procedure exists for negotiating the means of assessment with appropriate committees such as Boards of Study, Faculty Board.
- Identify student expectations.
- Check that expectations match overall course objectives.
- Identify linkages to other parts of the course.

COMPLIERS AND DESIGNERS

Consider:

- The subject matter involved.
- Structure and nature of the relevant course.
- General goals of the course and any specific learning objectives which may need to be written.
- Background and general quality of the students.
- Most efficient and effective method of setting the assessment.
- Most efficient and effective procedures for assessing.
- Value of meaningful, lasting learning enhanced by the experience of doing the assessment.
- Benefits to be gained by students having to reconsider information, values, skills acquired previously.

GUIDELINES FOR CLINICAL ASSESSMENTS

1. Set an assessment that will be useful to students in their future postings.
2. State the purpose of the assessment.
3. State the expected length of any report(s). (For example, number of words, length in pages) or duration of a practical or problem-solving exercise.
4. Identify any sections to a report.
5. Check that the time available for students to carry out the assessment is realistic.
6. Avoid an assessment where the students spend a long time on trivia.
7. Set an assessment that incorporates previous learning and extends experience.
8. Clearly state student expectations.
9. Provide assessor checklists or identify how the process will be conducted.

10. Identify detailed responses and reactions required from a simulated patient, active mannequin, or other equipment.
11. Compose a detailed marking procedure and state performance criteria for each sub-division.
12. Ensure the assessment with its mark scheme assesses an individual student at a pre-determined level.
13. Identify in detail the resources and equipment needed and what should not be available.
14. Provide a clear statement of assessment procedures to tutorial staff and to students.
15. Ensure all interested parties agree to procedure.

So far, most of what has been said relates to more formal assessment. The same principles apply to the assessment of staff in a training post. Such assessment is vital to signpost progress along what should be an agreed educational pathway.

At the beginning of the assessment period when trainer and trainee should hold full discussion to determine the present status and the trainees own expectations from the post. Indicators of progress should be mutually agreed within specified time limits and defined as learning objectives.

For example, a new doctor on a coronary care unit might be told, 'Within the next two weeks you will be able to demonstrate the knowledge and presentation skills necessary for you to act as a clinician on the cardiac arrest team.'

Or, a research fellow might hear, 'Within the next four weeks you will have written up your research findings and presented them in a format suitable for publication.' Obviously, assessments can be a mixture of the oral, written or observation techniques described here. The limits have been agreed at the outset, the parameters set, and the outcome is a very solid basis for a reference!

When assessments have been set up there is need for them to checked. A validation procedure such as the form overleaf could be used. Similar forms can be used for all types of assessment. Procedural guidelines are important and also can be used in tutor and examiner training courses. The training can be a one-day course focused on setting and marking procedures.

VALIDATION FORM

This form is designed to assist in the evaluation of the quality and suitability of the practical and clinical assessments.

Assessment title

Originator   Date

Validation panel   Date

This is the most suitable form of assessment   ❏ Yes ❏ No

This assessment meets all the guidelines   ❏ Yes ❏ No

Guidelines not met: 1 2 3 4 5 6 7 8 9 10 11 12 13 14 15

In the table below tick as appropriate:
*   1 no amendment*
*   2 minor amendment*
*   3 considerable amendment*

1. The assessment meets its purposes. 1 2 3
2. The instructions to students state the requirements clearly.
3. The assessment can only be completed with a
    depth of understanding. 1 2 3
4. The assessment can only be completed with a
    depth of commitment. 1 2 3
5. The time allocated for completion is reasonable. 1 2 3
6. The assessment is clear and unambiguous in its expectations. 1 2 3
7. The set of performance criteria relates well to the expectations. 1 2 3
8. The set of performance criteria relates well to the purposes
    of the assessment. 1 2 3
9. The performance criteria are at an appropriate level of difficulty. . . 1 2 3
10. The ideas, values, or skills being assessed are consistent
    with course objectives. 1 2 3
11. The assessment could promote questioning of the ideas,
    values and skills involved. 1 2 3

SUGGESTED FURTHER READING

Colliver, J. A., Vu, N. V. & Markwell, S. J., et al. (1991) – Reliability and efficiency of components of clinical competence assessed with five performance-based examinations using standardized patients. Medical Education, 25, 303-310

Cox, K. R. & Evans, C. E. (Ed.) (1988) – The Medical Teacher (2nd edition) Edinburgh, Churchill Livingstone. (Section 4 Assessment)

Cuschieri, A., Gleeson ,F. A. & Harden, R. M. (1979) – A new approach to a final examination in surgery. Use of the objective structured clinical examination. Annals of the Royal College of Surgeons of England 61, 400-405

Harden, R. McG. & Gleeson, F. (1979) – Assessment of clinical competence using objective structured clinical examination (OSCE) Medical Education 13, 41-51

Harris, D. & Bell, C. (1994) – Evaluating and Assessing for Learning (revised paper back edition) London, Kogan Page

Hart, I., Harden, R. McG. & Mulholland H. (Ed) (1991) – Approaches to the Assessment of Clinical Competence. (Proceedings of the 5th Ottawa Conference) Dundee

Keeves, J. P. (Ed.) (1988) – Educational Research, Methodology and Measurement: An International Handbook Oxford, Pergamon Press (Attitude Measurement pp 421-436; Measurement Theory (pp 241-330) including: criterion-referenced measurement; validity; reliability)

Keynan, A., Friedman M. & Benbassat, J. (1987) – Reliability of global rating scales in the assessment of clinical competence of medical students Medical Education, 21, 477-481

Kong, H.H.P., Neufield,V. & Hart I., et al. (1987) – Symposium: The Evaluation of Clinical Competence during Residency Training. Annals R.C.P.S.C. 20, 5, 361-366

Newble, D.I. (Ed.) (1989) – Guidelines for the development of effective and efficient procedures for the assessment of clinical competence in Wakeford, R. (Ed.) Proceedings of the Fourth Cambridge Conference on Medical education, Cambridge, Office of the Regius Professor of Physic, University of Cambridge

Newble, D.I. & Cannon, R. (1991) – A Handbook for Clinical Teachers. (2nd Edition). London, M.T.P. Press. (Chapter 6, Assessing the Student)

Newble D. I., Jolly B. C. & Wakeford, R. E. (Ed.) (1994) – The Certification and Re-Certification of Doctors: Issues in the Assessment of Clinical Competence. Cambridge, Cambridge University Press

Osler, W. Sir (1913) – Examinations, Examiners and Examinees. The Lancet Oct. 11 1913, 1047-1049

Rowntree, D. (1988) – Assessing Students: How Shall We Know Them? London, Kogan Page

Stevenson, Z.J. (1983) – Assessment of the Clinical Performance of Medical Students: a Survey of Methods. Office of Research and Development for education in Health Profession, University of North Carolina Medical School. Chapel Hill, N.C., USA

Stillman, P.L. (1992) – Normal Physical Examination Instructor's Manual Massachusetts, University of Massachusetts Medical Center

Van der Vleuten, C.P.M. & Swanson, D.B. (1990) – Assessment of clinical skills with standardised patients: state of the art Teaching and Learning in Medicine 2, 58-76

Williams, R.G., Barrons, H.S. & Vu, N.V. et al. (1978) – Direct, standardised assessment of clinical competence. Medical Education , 482-489

CHAPTER 6
Curriculum and Course Development

LYNNE PEYTON & RODNEY PEYTON

INTRODUCTION

THIS CHAPTER deals with the design and development of *curriculae* and courses. Both are essential at undergraduate and postgraduate levels, and provide the essential framework for professional development. By the very nature of the profession, the overall structure is predetermined and developed over a number of years. Once it is in position, the process of achieving the various aims and objectives, allows plenty of scope for a learner-centred approach. In other words, the outcomes are determined, but the process of achieving them is not.

As well as the six elements of design, the ten phases of curriculum development are detailed and discussed. The section concludes with a brief discussion of five different curriculum models.

Designing and developing a course is a very similar process to putting together a curriculum. It is discussed in that context. The concept of a grid covering subject areas and learning levels required in the various domains is outlined as a useful tool in the planning of a course.

THE DEFINITION OF CURRICULUM

The word 'curriculum' derives from the Latin *currere* meaning to run. This implies a sense of movement and direction and thus suggests the function of a curriculum is to provide a template or design for a specific learning process. It narrows the required fields of learning in terms of knowledge, skills and attitudes, identifies needs and sets goals for the learner. Essentially, the professional body controls these on society's behalf. They indicate how practitioners are expected to behave and what they are supposed to know. By necessity grounded in ethics, it specifies the subject area and the standards to be achieved and is thereby capable of being externally validated.

As the knowledge base of every field and topic within medicine is rapidly expanding, efficiency in the learning process is required to ensure some distillation of available information. In order to develop systematically to a point where they can be assessed as being competent, independent practitioner trainees also need clear direction and guidance. Although some propose an 'open' learner-centred approach with only the most general of guidelines, this would be extremely inefficient. In this era of high technology and constant change, the temptation to start with a blank sheet must be resisted. There is neither the time nor the need to re-invent the wheel. Trainees must understand what the wheel can do, reflect on its usefulness in the light of present day knowledge and determine new ways in which it can be evolved. Thus, the curriculum is more than a mere syllabus. It provides an essential framework for translating broadly based knowledge into an information base that can underpin action in the real world.

CURRICULAR CYCLE

The curricular cycle involves development through needs assessment, design, and implementation phases. After this, outcomes are reviewed and evaluated against the original needs assessment. Needs change with societal expectations. The emphasis on different aspects varies with the participants' and teachers' perceived needs. The dynamic curriculum requires change and resource management.

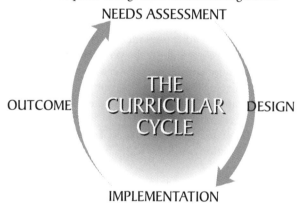

Fig. 1 THE CURRICULAR CYCLE

Needs assessment gives rise to the 'official' curriculum. This can be set out as an institutional prospectus providing overall purpose and content information. While

92

need assessment tells how the course is designed, many other factors and constraints have to be considered.

At the end of the day, a successful curriculum must achieve as close a match as possible between *official* and *functional* versions and outcome. There are three basic design imperatives:

- It must achieve the institutional requirements.
- It must be relevant and meaningful to the tutors who will inevitably have their own subject bias.
- It must meet the learners' personal goals as they develop and mature professionally.

93

Learning occurs during the implementation phase, usually through the provision of courses. These can be external courses such as distance learning or internal. An example of the latter would be on the job training or individual study. This is the active phase and represents the *functional* curriculum. Implementation may vary from heavily teacher-centred to more learner-centred. These overlap with, but vary from, the *official* curriculum by the very fact that individuals are involved. Finally, there is the outcome from the curricular process. This deals with what learning actually took place. Learners bring their background experience and perceptions of what is relevant in their 'real world'. Therefore, each has his or her own agenda making the process meaningful to each in a different way. Everyday working practice constraints including facilities, finance and manpower alter the perception of the materials presented and thus the translation of this knowledge into action. For this reason, formal evaluation is essential to set outcomes in the working practice context. They provide feedback to the needs assessment that influences the design process theory. In this way the curricular cycle closes.

CURRICULUM DEVELOPMENT

For any curriculum to remain relevant and maintain its quality standards there must be a continuing evolutionary process. This should be relatively slow and measured, since quick or spontaneous changes in direction can be very unsettling and cause uncertainty, especially for those charged with carrying it through.

The curriculum is meant to guide both teachers and learners. Adults respond best when they have internal motivation. This emotional state reflects the way past experience forms attitudes and values and gives rise to expectations. For the best outcomes, teachers must be committed to the content of their courses. No matter how rational certain changes may seem, attempts to force them through without co-operation inevitably leads to de-motivation and a less than optimal outcome. The curriculum must sit well with adult education principles. It must allow learners to reflect in the context of their own experience and uses a task or problem orientated approach. Objectives must be clear so that both teachers and learners judge performance with criterion based feedback.

Accordingly, the curriculum development process can be divided into ten phases following in a logical sequence. These are:

1. Needs assessment.
2. Setting a clear aim and goals.
3. Brainstorming ideas.

4. Identification of constraints.
5. Editing ideas to produce a formal list.
6. Identification of methods of assessment.
7. Setting timetables.
8. Curriculum publication.
9. Implementation.
10. Evaluation.

Each will be discussed in turn:

NEEDS ASSESSMENT

A curriculum rarely starts from scratch. Most develop from already existing schemes. They are altered in the light of policy development, research findings, new educational processes or on the basis of evaluation and feedback from learners, teachers and external agencies. The drive to alter the curriculum is particularly strong when outcomes evaluated in the practical situation show a mismatch between the written curriculum theory and the real world. Thus, it must be rooted in real practice and not perceived as 'ivory tower' idealism imposed from on high. It must direct without being unnecessarily prescriptive and there must be opportunities for creativity. Unforeseen outcomes may be equally valid. Nor must it be overly restrictive in teaching and learning methods.

Identifying what is worth learning is the purpose of needs analysis. It requires knowledge of the *status quo* so that the curriculum can be designed to develop and reinforce good practice by setting down the standards of performance. It is important that those responsible for curriculum development consult widely with academic institutions and those involved in awarding external qualifications, as well as with professional representatives, those in training and consumer interests. Afterwards, a curriculum development committee representing the interested parties considers the collated and analysed findings.

SETTING A CLEAR AIM AND GOALS

The committee determines the curriculum's overall aim and sets clear goals. Each must be specific, justified and defined within particular domains of learning. It can be relatively simple to define those goals that are attainable through the acquisition of knowledge and skills. It is much less easy to define those that depend on achieving interpersonal skills, motivation, or commitment. This encompasses the area of professional ethic. Once delineated, the general aim and goals need to be rigorously thought through by the committee in terms of face validation.

BRAINSTORMING IDEAS

To determine the breadth of the subject matter to be learned and understood there must be a brainstorming of ideas for each goal. This shapes the curriculum and underpins the development of a coherent plan. There will be many different elements. Some of these are linked readily while others are not so obviously related. During this phase, it is imperative to note all that is potentially relevant. This list must be analysed, edited, and correlated.

IDENTIFICATION OF CONSTRAINTS.

Possible constraints on the curriculum should be identified at the earliest possible opportunity. These may include bureaucratic constraints. Institutional rules and regulations, legislation, statute and government policy may all have a considerable impact. Budgetary constraints are inevitable. Limited availability of suitable venues or appropriate equipment may give rise to physical and timetable setting problems. Manpower issues such as service commitments limit both trainer availability and trainees' capacity to avail themselves of courses. The influence of personal ethics, principles, and preferences should not be underestimated.

EDITING IDEAS TO PRODUCE A FORMAL LIST

To provide a short-list of subjects and subject matter, ideas generated for each goal need to be collated and considered within the context of the constraints. After this, order these under subject headings and, where necessary, identify sequencing issues. Inevitably, this resembles a 'wish list' and hard decisions have to be made about which elements are essential and which non-essential. To keep the curriculum in line with both needs analysis and consultation process it is important to refer back to the consultation exercise findings. It must not revert to being based exclusively on the committee's ideas. To be marketable, the curriculum must address and be seen to address, the target population's identified needs and priorities.

IDENTIFICATION OF METHODS OF ASSESSMENT.

An integral part of the curriculum development is agreement on the assessment methods to be used and whether these are to be internal or external. The way assessment is carried out influences both the teacher's and learner's perception of the value of the course. To a large extent, it will drive the teaching and learning process and thus determine how the subject will be taught. Congruity between the curriculum philosophy and the assessment process is essential.

For instance, in a curriculum heavily orientated towards task centred and problem solving approaches, the outcomes could not be fully assessed by a multiple choice question paper. Workplace assessment techniques or the use of practical scenarios as outlined in Chapter Five are more appropriate.

SETTING TIMETABLES.

Ideally, the timetable represents a coherent curriculum plan. It starts on a 'macro' level looking at the introduction or revisiting of particular subject blocks throughout a long programme. Later at the 'micro' level it details the shape and context of a particular day or week. Once this is accomplished, the curriculum has substance. Aims and goals are explicit, the priorities of subjects to be covered are determined, the methods of assessment specified and the outline of a timetable for delivery established.

CURRICULUM PUBLICATION

Time permitting, key stakeholder representatives should assess the draft curriculum. These should include some of those who participated in the original needs assessment. Fine tuning will be based on their responses. Market testing is crucial for all but the most established and financially viable *curriculae*. In all other circumstances, attempting to determine both market appeal and ultimate viability is wise. Among the numerous options for doing this, are obtaining initial course sponsorship or determining the demand for places through advertising. In order to determine the likelihood of hospital or community trusts taking up a number of places more direct approaches can be made.

IMPLEMENTATION

Implementation may involve a pilot scheme to test some or all of the new elements before introducing them wholesale into the curriculum. It must be carefully managed. Wherever possible, pilot new elements to iron out unforeseen difficulties arising from translating theory into reality. A pilot scheme best uses limited resources to determine the most effective content, sequencing, delivery mechanisms and assessment techniques.

EVALUATION

Evaluation must be ongoing and carried out using as many different methods as possible. It should look at all aspects of any proposed change, to determine whether what the planning committee perceived as a method of addressing the needs, identified initially, has had the desired affect. This process of determining value is more fully described in Chapter Ten.

CURRICULUM DESIGN

Curriculum design involves ordering the planning exercise results and putting them into sequence. It is the intermediate step between taking *what* has to be learned and translating it into *how* it is to be learned. It also allows management of the process. This section deals with design phase elements, the style or styles envisaged and different curriculum plan structures.

The Elements

The six elements to be considered address fundamental questions on the content of the course and how it is to be managed.

1. Subject Matter
2. Outcomes
3. Student Knowledge Base
4. Constraints
5. Assessment Methods
6. Evaluation.

SUBJECT MATTER

Subject matter derives from the aim and objectives decided during the curriculum development phase. It must be teased out and subdivided into the various learning domains and the levels expected within each. For example, does the curriculum simply require an understanding of some knowledge or does it demand an ability to evaluate knowledge in the light of experience?

OUTCOMES

Each domain's expected outcomes should specify knowledge levels, competence demonstrated or the ability for professional reflection. Priorities should be set. At the top of the scale, content should be graded in terms of what *must* be known or demonstrated. In the middle it should concern itself with what *should* be known or demonstrated. At the bottom comes what constitutes desirable but not essential information. This part of the process requires practitioners' active involvement to ensure practical working environment decisions have priority and that decisions are not left to academics, educators and other specialists. However, the assistance of these same academics, educators and other specialists is vital in constructing the design.

STUDENT KNOWLEDGE BASE

This looks at the learners' characteristics, particularly their level of background and previous knowledge. Assessing whether they are all on a similar level is important and may require pre-tests to estimate what they actually know as opposed to what they state they know on an application form.

Obviously, designing a curriculum is easier when learners have a common knowledge base or similar experiences. For instance, when designing higher specialist training. However, there may be many instances when a mixed group with varying experiences and expertise, perhaps even across specialities, is quite acceptable. This gives trainees the opportunity to learn from each other's experience in different fields. An example might be a Training the Trainers course or a management development programme. In such diverse groups, both the seconders of participants and course participants themselves have their own agendas. These have an obvious impact on the outcomes.

Very early on, the trainees' wants should be matched to their perceived needs. Compromises should be sought to develop agreed achievable outcomes in spite of divergent knowledge bases and expectations.

CONSTRAINTS

Curriculum design constraints and their likely impact on the process need to be identified from the outset. These may be concerned with financial or human resources, especially any of the tutors' potential training needs. There may well be particular professional or governmental regulations that, coupled with ethical issues, might have an impact on the way a course is run. Such an instance may be patients' involvement. The final schedule has to be convenient for staff, for other courses running concurrently or with particular service commitments. Time devoted to promotion of the course of study may be needed.

All these issues must be addressed for proper management of process and outcomes. If authority can be delegated as locally as possible, control of curriculum design is enhanced. However, some obvious problems arise if such delegation is passed too far down the line. For example, those with local responsibility may lobby for their own agenda. They may not be motivated to drive the overall curriculum. They may be loathe to compromise if they recognise potential loss of kudos or income or if a cutback in their sphere of influence is agreed. On the other hand, one particularly powerful individual may manage to overshadow others either by force of personality and/or his 'past history' among the group. Such individuals often have disproportionate influence and upset the group's balance and hence the curriculum.

Those involved in the design process must subscribe to a common aim, work backwards to determine the appropriate nature and level of contribution from individual providers and decide how these can best be co-ordinated. Perhaps, embodied in an early mission statement, this reinforces the need for agreed aims and clear goals.

ASSESSMENT METHODS

Assessment methods influence outcomes. Therefore they need to be agreed on early in the design process. Is it to be managed internally or externally? How detailed will these assessments be and what are the most appropriate methods to use? Any course outcome is assessment-driven since this influences student perception of what is important. This varies with the style or process adopted. If examinations are based on factual knowledge, inevitably students cram facts beforehand. This leads to superficial learning, even though the course may be based on a deeper problem-solving approach. Assessment methods should reflect any intention of directing students into a problem-solving mode and require a demonstration of analytical skills.

EVALUATION

Finally, the design needs to be evaluated in the light of experience. This is vital to ensure that the curriculum in action is capable of delivering the agreed aims and goals. (See Chapter Four.)

CURRICULUM STYLE

This deals with the curriculum's internal structure. Numerous generalisations can be made about curriculum design. In the first method, based on feedback either from participants or through research into outcomes, modifications are made to an existing design. To take into account a perceived deficit, parts of the curriculum are altered. Evaluation is carried out to judge whether the change produced the desired outcome.

Another technique involves starting from scratch once the required knowledge base is determined, providing links between the various strands to integrate the information. That accomplished, translate it into the practical situation. A third method takes the practical situation as its starting point. It looks at various practical problems and works backwards identifying skills and the knowledge base required in order to solve particular problems.

Each of these must begin with a clear statement of expected outcome and work out the best method to achieve it. An obvious drawback is that the whole learning process becomes geared towards pre-selected outcomes and fails to acknowledge the value of unintended conclusions however appropriate they may be. The system regards these as deviations from the intended path and does not grant them any intrinsic value. In this way, imaginative and opportunistic experiences may be lost or languish without being exploited to their full potential. In an environment that encourages reflection on practice such unintended learning outcomes can be as valuable as those anticipated from an 'official' curriculum.

Finally, at the other end of the spectrum, a curriculum may be designed without specifically defined outcomes but with indicated general lines of direction. Any movement along a particular path is acceptable in this situation. Results derive from the learner's creative and unstructured approach.

The curriculum should expand the knowledge base, maintain interest, provide or facilitate acquisition of knowledge relevant to practice and encourage creativity and analytical skills. Therefore, it is apparent that no one route is correct. Different people at different times learn most effectively from one or other method. It all depends on the subject matter to be learned and current constraints.

CURRICULUM STRUCTURE

There are five types of structure:

1. Vertical
2. Horizontal
3. Spiral
4. Web
5. Core plus Options.

The appropriateness of each depends on a number of factors. In deciding on a particular model, objectives should be studied closely and any links established.

VERTICAL

If the links are tenuous, a vertical or linear structure is most appropriate. Each piece of information or subject matter follows what went before in a sequential manner. It does not allow for concurrent activity. In consequence, the process may be very time consuming.

HORIZONTAL

It is best to try to establish links between different subjects, especially if these are fairly simple and obvious. The design reflects concurrent activity on a number of different subject areas. Linkage takes place later.

SPIRAL

Initially, the spiral curriculum deals with each subject at a fairly simple level. However, enough of the subject matter is covered to allow a natural progression and to provide a framework for advances in that particular subject when it is revisited. Early links established between all subjects are maintained, as they become more complex.

This sort of curriculum is complicated, time consuming and requiring of considerable co-operation between those delivering different subjects. Difficulties arise if they get out of sequence. For example, this happens when environmental or human resource problems prevent a particular subject area being taught in its allotted space. One teacher or tutor having overall responsibility for the curriculum, can overcome this problem. While such a situation may exist at first, it is unlikely to exist over the long term since one individual would need a very wide range of knowledge and expertise. In any case, trainees benefit from different tutors bringing different perceptions to the process.

WEB

In the web model, a number of subject areas are available simultaneously and it is up to the learner to decide which one to visit and when. This model is particularly attractive to mature, experienced and self motivated learners who have the ability to both choose subjects and determine how much depth to go into, dependent on circum-

99

stances at the time. This fits very well with a problem-based approach. The process has to be overseen quite closely with inexperienced learners. However, as they develop problem-based learning skills and can reflect on what they have learned, tutors can reduce their role and become facilitators.

CORE PLUS OPTIONS

The core plus options model implies that learners do not need to explore all subject areas but have to undertake certain core areas. After this, they are free to choose from a range of options that reflect other areas of interest and determine the subject matter's relevance to them at a particular time. This indicates the learner's need to achieve a prescribed level in specific subject areas along with options for further study in relevant areas. Arranging this can be hard since some options may be unpopular and poorly supported while others may be oversubscribed. Although, adult learners find this particularly attractive it leads to resource managing difficulties. The fit between the options offered and those in demand can be improved by effective need assessment. Flexibility achieved through co-operation with other institutions, offers low demand options.

This particular format differs from the other four. It fits within the other options to give them a degree of flexibility.

CONCLUSION

Curriculum design is fundamentally a question of looking at course content, its delivery, and the balance of analytical and creative activities. On this basis and, depending on the links between the various subjects, one chooses the most appropriate structure. It requires a critical path to order and sequence material and when agreeing timings to take into account relevant deadlines. Overall, the design must be changeable in the light of considered experience and evidenced deficiencies. Evolution rather than revolution best achieve designs.

Depending on the curriculum, one short course fulfils some. Others require a number of courses or independent study periods. In the former case, the curriculum gives a template for the course. In the latter, the information to be delivered should be broken up into manageable proportions requiring objectives, outcomes and a method of delivery. Therefore, for any curriculum there will be more than one study method or programme capable of delivering the learning experience. The goal is to find the most effective and efficient way of connecting the subjects, learners, teachers, and resources.

COURSE DESIGN

A course is the practical mechanism that delivers the curriculum, the curriculum in action. It can be defined as a group of learning events, linked by a common theme, run in a particular sequence and for a finite amount of time. To give clear direction as to appropriate learning domains, both teaching methods and course assessment needs to be determined right at the outset.

Course and curriculum design is very similar. The starting point is to define the purpose of the course. Is it to stand alone, being set up to address one particular objective? Is it being run in conjunction with other courses to achieve a particular curriculum? Once the purpose is determined it can be translated into terms of expected outcomes. In particular, this shows how the course will benefit the participants' educational needs.

Once subjects and potential assessment techniques are decided, a brainstorming session determines individual topics within each area. The list generated should be as comprehensive as possible. From this a short list of topics emerges. This includes those clearly grounded in practice and most appropriate. A final checking of the curriculum's stated intentions and the outcome of any needs analysis ensures that the appropriate direction is maintained with particular attention being paid to boundaries and other constraints.

At this time, a grid to set an overall structure is useful. Topics are listed to the side. Split into levels of hierarchy, the domains are placed along the top. Various intersections of subject matter versus levels should be ticked or filled-in so the overall pattern of the course becomes evident at a glance. (See figure 2.)

		DOMAIN									
		Cognitive			Psychomotor			Affective			Inter-Personal	
		1&2	3	4&5	1&2	3	4&5	1&2	3	4&5	Task	Process
	Patient Selection			✓				✓				✓
	Set Up In Theatre		✓				✓				✓	
	Insertion Of Ports	✓					✓					
	Diathermy Safety		✓				✓			✓		
	Operative Cholangiogram	✓				✓		✓				

Fig. 2 A GRID TO HELP IN PLANNING A LAPAROSCOPIC CHOLECYSTECTOMY COURSE

The domains are as listed in Chapter Four. Each is divided into three zones for easy reference. *For instance, affective 1 = receive and 5 = acts.* Some of the course topics are listed on the left and suggested levels within the domains are marked with a tick. A glance at the grid indicates the expected outcomes and guides the course organiser towards the most appropriate teaching method. For instance, diathermy safety requires knowledge of theatre safety rules. As well, it may require an open discussion period in order to look at the affective domain's higher levels. Demonstration can teach the theatre set up. However, the learner must carry this out in a practical situation. He or she must instruct the operating staff on such points as leads positions and insufflator use. Instructing the camera operator must not be forgotten. The listing for operative cholangiogram implies that the learner only needs an understanding of how this is carried out but no requirement to personally perform the procedure.

The matrix helps structure the various learning and teaching activities.

More detailed information on individual participants is required. Generalisations can be made in the curriculum design stage. However, a course must be designed to fit in with participants' competence and perceived range of abilities to ensure it remains relevant to each. Everyone learns differently. Some respond best to heavily guided experiences. Others want to freely explore serialistic or holistic approaches. All must be allowed to relate the knowledge gained to their own experience.

Aristotle suggested that wisdom is the result of reflection on experience. While this basic tenet holds true it has to be adapted in this technological age, where wisdom might be defined as the ability to integrate new knowledge and then reflect on experience. Course organisers and tutors must be aware of each learner's motivation and whether it is externally or internally driven or both. Motivation determines whether learning is likely to be superficial or deep although maintenance of interest and knowledge or skills retention must be taken into account.

Once the participants' needs and the structure of the topics have been identified, the course can take shape. Time is one of the most critical factors and, working backwards from the end point, a critical path should be set to provide the framework within which learning events can be logically developed.

Other timetable constraints may be obvious from a study of the grid. Access to equipment or resources such as laboratories, ward or theatre space dictates when to schedule particular topics. The availability of specific teachers is usually critical and should be checked well in advance especially if they are practitioners with service commitments.

Students learn by individual study, from other students and from their teachers. The timetable should allow private study and various group interactions. Sufficient quantities of appropriate resource materials must be ready at the appropriate time. The course's logistics may need considerable organisation. In order to run smoothly, it requires a facilitator who understands the direction and outcome required and is able to make corrections during the course. Assessment methods for a course running for any length of time should be both formative and summative. Teaching is responsive to the learning process. Possible assessment methods are discussed more fully in Chapter Five.

Constraints

The time available for the course has already been discussed. However, finance is usually one of the biggest constraints on any course. Courses must not just be practical but financially feasible. The likely income is set against expenditure on items such as hiring equipment or lecture facilities, staff costs and payments to tutors including travel and accommodation. Faculty must be chosen for teaching ability as well as expertise. Clinical experts are not necessarily the best people to impart knowledge concisely and cogently. They may require direction and faculty training prior to the course.

In adult education, open discussion identifies problems and hidden agendas. It lets learners explore new information. They can compare this to their own and their peers' and experienced practitioners' past experience. Teachers may need help in developing the skill to facilitate and manage this dialogue constructively.

When learning in any professional context, observation of skilled practitioners and role modelling can help enliven the theoretical concepts. This is most obvious with problem solving techniques where learners observe skilled practitioners and their own peers solving workplace problems. In the early phases of developing professionalism, students usually need continual guidance.

At the outset, this may involve purely receptive learning and strong teacher-directed input. As learners develop and gain experience, they become more independent as practitioners and must be encouraged to reflect on their own practice. They must actively search for answers to problems by whatever means most suited to them. They achieve professional autonomy when they can do this. Teachers must act as facilitators in this process and must know how and by what means to decrease learner dependency. If, by the end of a course, learners are unable to use information to alter their practice, the course has failed them. No matter how efficient, concise and well organised a didactic course may appear, it must be evaluated by its learning outcomes. Ultimately, this is the only way to measure its usefulness.

Delivery Mode

On the job training, one of the best methods of keeping theory relevant to work practice, should make it easier for knowledge to be assimilated. However, work commitments have to be managed so that they do not impinge on teaching time. Also, the working environment may tire or stress learners so they have a less than optimal learning experience.

Day release or night classes can represent a compromise. However they are very tiring. A two to three days every few weeks block release takes learners out of their working environment and may greatly increase the capacity to learn and retain the information. It has the added advantage that information gained can be put to practical use within a very short time. The next meeting can be used to reflect on the usefulness of the last block of learning in the practical situation.

Sharing different perspectives is one of the obvious benefits of sharing experiences within a group. This phase may take up half to one day of a block release. The following days can be used to set up future projects based on previous work or on taking knowledge in a new direction. Using a block release is one of the more effective forms of distance learning. Learners have access to materials in their home environment and are encouraged to work at their own pace. Given the tendency for time scales to slip, the provision of dedicated time to study blocks enhances compliance with the schedule for the rest of the course.

The final model is a course run on a continuous or full time basis. This is usually most efficient for those working for higher qualifications such as degrees. It allows multiple courses to be combined with links between them as appropriate. The main disadvantage is that there are obvious financial implications not just for the course organisers but for those attending. They may be penalised in terms of finance or promotion because they have stopped work. Such courses tend to concentrate on theory and fail to achieve an appropriate balance between that and practice.

In conclusion, the process of course design is similar to that of curriculum design but should be more learner-centred. It should focus on both the learner's needs and on the practical applications of the subject matter. The nature of the learning that takes place is closely linked to the assessment method. In turn, this must reflect the intended outcomes.

PUTTING THIS CHAPTER INTO ACTION

There are many similarities between curriculum and course development which are drawn out in this chapter. The process can be summed up in the 5 Ds.

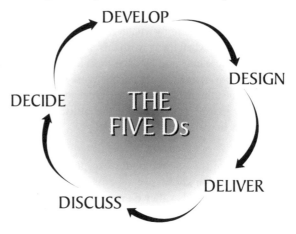

Fig. 3   THE FIVE Ds

Constant development keeps the curriculum or the course relevant and maintains its standards. Undue haste at this phase can be counter-productive. A slow measured approach is recommended. Ample time must be taken to discuss the assessment of need and the provision of clear aims and goals.

The design must take on the aim and goals from the development phase *and* look closely at the subject matter and intended outcomes. A detailed analysis of the learners' background and time constraints, finance or other resources is required. Since assessment is recognised as one of the most basic learning process drives this must be addressed and agreed at the outset. When determining the basic curriculum, the links between various subjects and the subject matter itself must be studied. The main models are the vertical, horizontal, spiral, web or core plus options.

A grid showing subjects against the learning domains allows links to be determined at a glance. This helps to construct an overall course shape and assists the selection of an appropriate mode of delivery. Workplace training, day or block release options, distance learning or full time attendance, all have benefits and drawbacks. The most appropriate model is determined after considering learners' needs, teachers' requirements and subject matter.

SUGGESTED FURTHER READING

Bines H. & Watts D. (1992) – Developing Professional Education: A Polytechnic Perspective. Open University Press. Buckingham

Entwhistle N.J. et al (1990) – Handbook of Educational Ideas and Practices. Routledge. London

Harden R.M. (1986) – Approaches to Curriculum Planning Medical Education 20 (458-466)

Romiszoski A.J. (1977) – Designing Instructional Systems. Kogan Page Ltd. London

Rowntree D. (1985) – Developing Courses for Students; Paul Chapman Publishers Ltd. London

Unruh G.G. & Unruh A. (1984) – Curriculum Development, Process & Progress; McCutcheon, New York

Walker D.F. & Soltis J.F. (1986) – Curriculum And Aims; Teacher College Press, New York

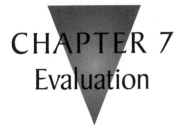

CHAPTER 7
Evaluation

BRIAN JOLLY & RODNEY PEYTON

INTRODUCTION

THIS CHAPTER FOCUSES on course evaluation, rationale and methodology, and examines stakeholder inter-relationships. This includes academic and professional institutions, faculty and course tutors, and employers seconding the trainees as well as all those using the service.

It describes the three basic elements of evaluation and then poses five fundamental questions. Why? What? Who? When? How? The chapter concludes by listing the ten steps of evaluation.

THE EVALUATION CYCLE

Like other professions, medicine is experiencing an accelerating rate of change, largely as a result of technological advances, drug treatments and ever increasing public expectations. Consequently, the profession has a responsibility to analyse change and a need to influence its pace and direction. This responsibility should be readily embraced, rather than resisted or feared. The medical educators' role is to ensure that training keeps pace with developments and remains relevant to clinical practice and to societal expectations. Evaluation is crucial and ongoing, forming part of a continuous cycle of needs assessment, course design, delivery, evaluation and feedback.

Evaluation at primary and secondary level in education usually means assessing individuals' levels of achievement against educational objectives set in advance. These tend to be summative and allow individuals to be compared with others in the peer group. (See Chapter Five.) However, these checks tend to be bureaucratic and formal with a precise end point such as attaining a grade. Adults who become much more diverse in what and how they learn as they progress in their chosen career find such rigidity very restrictive.

Any profession is more than science, it is also an art. How decisions are arrived at and communicated in practical situations may be as important as their scientific basis. Thus, measurement of professional growth has to be qualitative as well as quantitative. This makes it difficult to lay down a specific end point for all learning and indeed it is inappropriate to do so. The individual and the community must determine whether the process benefits both parties, in other words has some intrinsic value.

It is not enough that learners enjoyed the process, or even that learning occurred. Rather, it is important that new behaviours are of practical significance in the normal working environment and, at the end of the day, have some effect on the community, for instance, by improving patient outcomes. It is notable that though learners may have disliked what they saw as a difficult and challenging process, the desired improvement in patient outcome was achieved.

In order to carry out the process properly, the evaluators, the learners involved, the techniques to be used and the general evaluation environment must be considered. Evaluators need to know the correct judging standard. It is best that these are peripheral to the main thrust, keeping personal bias as low as possible. Major stakeholders tend to be in managerial positions, have financial or political involvement, and be educational institutions and their teaching staff and other providers. The latter must participate willingly and recognise that evaluation can help them to reflect, develop, and grow as teachers.

Sometimes after an evaluation has taken place the findings suggest that change is inevitable. Initially, this may be uncomfortable for those who have reached a fairly autonomous stage in their careers, especially if they feel the process is being imposed on them. Professional colleagues and management must be supportive and help provide the environment conducive to experimentation and change. All participants should have confidence in the outcomes, recognising them as both valid and useful. If not, they are liable to resist or ignore them.

EVALUATION ELEMENTS

There are three basic elements to evaluation:

1. Information collection
2. The interpretation of that information
3. Making value judgements about progress and benefits to the target group.

Collection methods may be open or closed. In the closed method, questions are clearly defined. This is efficient from a financial and personnel standpoint but the outcomes are likely to be somewhat predetermined and restrictive since such techniques only answer the questions asked and do not allow for unintended, perhaps equally important, outcomes.

Open techniques widen the field of enquiry but have increased implications in financial, time and resources terms and there is much more scope for individual bias both in collecting and interpreting results. Thus, ensuing judgements depend heavily on collection methods and the interpretations placed on them. They must take into account the development context, the inputs and how the outcomes were achieved.

By definition, evaluation is the judging of an educational process or course in order to guide future direction. One gathers and interprets as much information about context, design, delivery, and outcomes as feasible.

WHY EVALUATE?

The only certainty about any course or curriculum is that to maintain relevance, it has to evolve with experience. Course and curriculum design is a dynamic process guided by the extent to which it meets the profession's and society's needs. To obtain appropriate information and to act on it, participants at all management levels must accept evaluation. Standing to benefit from greater expertise and higher standards, society must provide the finance.

Therefore, evaluation is vital in course development's cyclical change. It pilots, implements, evaluates, and feeds back into the developmental process. This gives indications for future investment and resource use and helps in developing appropriate actions to improve the product.

If all those involved understand that the intention is to improve the quality of the process and the product rather than simply provide a critique of individual or group performance, maximum co-operation should be achievable. It should be obvious that complacency does not belong in any ongoing course. The expectation is that change should and will occur. The evaluation process determines the degree and direction of change. The intention is to make it a positive experience as far as possible.

A well-planned evaluation produces broad-based understanding of the present position in terms of learners and learning. This allows for comparisons against agreed and uniform outcomes within and between institutions offering similar courses. It is essential to the overall stakeholders and allows any problems, real or perceived, to be identified and addressed. Confidence in 'the system's' quality assurance is vital since financial constraints and perceived value for money top the agenda. Validation of independent training outcomes, can be a very positive negotiating tool in procuring funds to sustain existing programmes and secure revenue for future training, developments and research.

WHAT SHOULD BE EVALUATED?

The entire design, piloting and implementation of a training programme may be evaluated from the first step of setting overall learning objectives to the actual teaching.

The fundamental questions are:
- What was the intended learning outcome?
- Was it appropriate?
- Was it achievable?
- How efficient and effective was the process?

The overall aims of the course of instruction must be looked at in terms of its likely effect on patient care. Even if a course is popular with participants and tutors it is inappropriate, if learning objectives were not readily transferable to the working environment. A classic example would be the participants in a course on laparoscopic bowel anastomosis returning to a hospital or unit where the equipment to carry out the procedure was unavailable.

Therefore, the design process must be assessed to determine whether the intended earning outcomes are valid in terms of the course's overall aims, workplace appropriateness and the particular group of learners. Can it deliver appropriate teaching in terms of knowledge, skills, and attitudes? Does it fit well with adult education principles by using appropriate styles to foster the desire to learn?

Well evaluated pilot programmes can be immensely important to the final product. To be valuable, it must be sufficiently similar to the main programme to enable valid conclusions and hence course modification to be made.

In evaluating successful course implementation, the following should be considered:

- Is there internal consistency between the various elements?
- Are the teaching methods and materials appropriate?
- Were the learning objectives specified for each element?
- Was sufficient time given for the outcomes to be achieved and assessed?
- How satisfactory was the process to both students and faculty?
- Was the environment appropriate? Variations in temperature or lighting, distractions such as noise (including on call bleeps and telephones) can disrupt an otherwise carefully designed and well thought out programme.
- Did the tutor and students set ground rules in advance to minimise interruptions?
- Were the design and delivery cost-efficient and was the course properly resourced?
- Were the outcomes such as to warrant further financial investment?

WHO SHOULD EVALUATE?

All those with a significant interest in course development should have input into what issues should be reviewed. They have the power to promote or undermine and must be represented to ensure ownership of outcomes and their commitment to any proposed plan. Finding this ownership and inherent responsibility concept foreign, some stakeholders may be difficult to engage and thus feel threatened by any suggestion they should actively participate. Each is likely to have his or her own agenda. This may or may not fit well with the common aims of the course, especially if any party feels press ganged into taking part. Many who are quite prepared to criticise will not participate in debate or proffer solutions.

A small steering group is ideally suited to the careful thought and planning evaluation requires. As it proceeds, this group must look at results in terms of the experience being gained. Group members must be flexible in their approach since unintended outcomes may be some of the programme's most valuable consequences.

The steering group's pivotal role and authority should be a consequence of its cross sectional representation of interested parties that range from fundholders to college faculty, from course providers to professional providers not to mention the students themselves. This group guides and directs evaluation down to an individual level and produces recommendations with implications for future practice. In general terms, the steering group's role can be seen as determining:

- Remit
- Boundaries
- Time-scales
- Sample size
- Methodologies
- Nature of the evaluation
- Type of report.

WHEN SHOULD EVALUATION BE CARRIED OUT?

Evaluation is intrinsic to each step of every programme. Therefore, it should take place before, during and after the programme. Prior to the course, the programme should be assessed in the light of overall aims and goals. Teaching and learning objectives should match as closely as possible the learners' wants and needs. The programme must have face validity. This means it must appear to be a reasonable method of setting about the various tasks in terms of knowledge, skills and attitudes and environmental or financial constraints. The course must appear feasible, provide a useful learning experience easily translatable to the workplace, and be carried out in a manner consistent with adult education principles.

Evaluation within a course is valuable if it is scheduled for more than two or three days. An internal steering group representing participants, faculty and administration allows for constant adjustment of content in the light of developing experience. Such ongoing, formative evaluations enhance the course's potential in terms of process and relevance of outcomes.

As long as facilitators adhere to overall aims and guidelines the longer the course, the greater its flexibility. Learners and the trainers should have the opportunity to get course organisers' and even external steering group feedback. This can take place during a protracted course, or immediately after a short one. Feedback may be formal or informal. The latter might involve sharing test results or, as part of mentoring arrangements, discussions with trainees. Time must be devoted to similar activities at the end of the course. In order to be of maximum influence, these should be scheduled and structured formal tests or discussions. Feedback needs careful handling and might involve sharp and focused five to ten minute episodes during the course and thirty minutes at the end.

Afterwards, when there has been time to translate the learned activities into work practice, further evaluation is necessary to demonstrate the long-term benefits of the course.

- Did it have the desired effect?
- If not, what would make it more successful?
- Were both the needs and the wants of the participants satisfactorily aligned and addressed?

111

Examining before, during, and after the programme provides a wealth of information. Evaluation's strength is in its use of varying approaches and techniques. Both qualitative and quantitative methods contribute to developing an overall picture of the programme and assessment of its future potential.

HOW TO EVALUATE

First define the evaluation's purpose. It is rare that one person makes this decision since stakeholders must be privy to any discussion. All participants must agree on major points at the outset. Unforeseen outcomes must always be allowed for since these may be very positive. It should be possible to fine-tune the evaluation purposes if an opportunity presents itself. At the very beginning, it is important to specify those with access to the results so that the process can be carried out in an atmosphere of mutual trust at all levels. Hence, the proffered information is likely to be accurate. Subsequent plans formulated on the basis of the evaluation are liable to be valid. A team approach is essential.

Evaluation considers course or curriculum process and outcomes and especially, the changes in the learners, or the value added by the various inputs. To determine this, define the state of knowledge or skill before the educational intervention and use this as a baseline against which to evaluate change and determine whether it is in the 'desired' direction.

Once outcomes are determined, evaluation methods can be matched to what is to be evaluated. Objective methods such as questionnaires, surveys, and test results work best when one can define objectives and end points, most obviously when dealing with skills and competencies. Qualitative methods are more relevant when objectives are more open ended. An example might be where much of the course involves problem-solving activities or where process issues are important. If a highly structured approach with pre-planned objectives lending themselves to quantitative data is over emphasised, issues such as programme quality are likely to be neglected. While such quantitative approaches may address planners' and administrators' anticipated results, they tend to restrict and limit. They are unlikely to provide insight into the nature and character of the course or to the interactions that occurred.

Conversely, more open techniques such as unstructured observation and interviews, reflect the group dynamics but can be very time consuming. One must strike a balance between the two to find a combination appropriate to each particular exercise.

Potential information sources include students, faculty, organisers and the institution or governing body, all of whom bring to bear individual biases in terms of their expectations of the course. Evaluators must try to remain impartial and objective. Use third party observers where possible or identify as information gatherers, particular session evaluators who lack vested interests. Such individuals might be tutors for different subjects on the same course or colleagues from another faculty. He or she should be able to assess consistency within course design and delivery. This is important since inconsistencies giving mixed messages on a topic during basic courses are not a good idea. Credibility is needed and course organisers should be known to practice what they preach.

There are many and varied evaluation methods each with strengths and weaknesses. They should be chosen for ease of use, analysing methods and data presentation, objectivity, reliability, sensitivity to issues and, not least, the time and effort required to carry them through. However, all need to be set against the potential payoff from the analyses of the information obtained.

There are three basic methods, observation, oral or written:

OBSERVATION METHODS

These may employ the participants themselves, including both faculty and students, or a third party. Video recording, another method, also captures performance or interactions for later analysis. All methods can distract both teachers and learners, alter normal dynamics and introduce a degree of artificiality. A third party's direct observation may not be cost efficient.

Further, observation such as this can be intrusive and put pressure on individuals. In such cases, both teachers and students feel under constant scrutiny and inevitably alter their normal behaviour. Only a sensitive approach in a supportive and agreed environment of mutual trust minimises these problems and helps observation become less obtrusive. This is important, since all should feel free to perform and give candid opinions during and after the formal learning experience. By taking care, results are not biased either by hostility or an overly collaborative response to the observer. If used properly, direct and indirect observational methods offer some of the best opportunities for individual self-analysis. This leads to improved performance and enhanced outcomes.

ORAL METHODS

The difficulty in structuring oral methods can actually be an advantage. First the difficulties. Individual interviews and group discussions are time consuming. Closed interviews and focussed discussions often lead to stilted and artificial communication and create tensions if issues important to one of the participants are dismissed or disregarded as irrelevant. The advantage is that information gained from more open-ended interventions or discussions can be wide ranging. It may uncover issues not previously considered by those arranging the evaluation, and may give extremely important insights into the workings of a course.

Frequently, these relate to hard to quantify quality issues and their full sense may not be easily analysed. For instance, it is difficult to weigh a particularly vociferous or opinionated individual's opinions. Others who have not had the opportunity to comment may or may not share them. To overcome these problems, group discussions have to be well facilitated and reporting must fairly represent the opinions expressed. Clearly, the evaluator needs good interpersonal skills and an ability to manage and report the group process.

WRITTEN METHODS

More structured written methods are commonly employed because they do not initially require a lot of evaluation. Seen as easy to use, they may be used in inappropriate circumstances. Part of that ease is that questionnaires, surveys and test reports may be quantified, making computer analysis and subsequent presentation of data more straightforward. However, generally, questionnaires tightly constructed to match programme objectives only reveal answers to those questions. Thus, these are thought out before hand and are insensitive to unidentified issues. Leaving space for 'comments' may offset this. However, in these instances comments are inclined to be short, sometimes cryptic, and do not lend themselves to in-depth analyses. The questionnaire is designed to test whether *prospecti*, course descriptors, handouts, or students records including log books and diaries are in keeping with the course syllabus.

Again, this may yield valuable information but usually it only gives the most general overview. Examination of records, logs and diaries may be more valuable if it is a prelude to a discussion. Specifically, a discussion teases out in greater detail particular 'critical incidents' occurring during the educational episode.

Once the information has been gathered, some form of value judgement must be made. The outcome, set against the initial intentions of course or curriculum, allows assessment as to its utility in process and outcome. However, before implementing changes based on the evaluation, the validity and reliability of the information needs to be determined. Are the results reproducible? What would happen if the course had a different student or faculty mix? Did the evaluation methods cause any side effects? Were methods diverse enough to look at all the important issues? Were there ripple effects, such as problems with peer relations or amongst hierarchies, unique to this group? Given the constraints on the procedure's value can the results and recommendations be regarded as sufficiently robust to support course or curriculum change?

To complete the cycle, any more than a slight tinkering needs of itself to be evaluated on future occasions, hopefully continuing an upward spiral of quality and effectiveness.

PUTTING THIS CHAPTER INTO ACTION

Evaluation, an active, cyclical process judges the merit of an education programme or process by gathering information about it from as wide a perspective as possible so that decisions about change can be made. In general terms that information should be specific and quantifiable.

It is important to understand that evaluation is not simply a 'learner satisfaction' indicator although this is, of course, of importance. Rather, evaluation looks at the links between goals, aims and objectives of a course and the eventual outcome. It should look, as widely as possible, at all the issues involved and consider the process as well as the end point.

The evaluation cycle involves ten steps. These are very similar to those in clinical research and audit:

1. List the aims and objectives of the course.
2. Find out at whom the course is aimed, their present level of knowledge, understanding or skill and determine their needs.
3. Decide if the course is appropriate to those needs (face validity).
4. Consider which issues should be addressed and therefore the constitution of a representative steering group.

5. Discuss and agree with the group those specific aspects that are to be evaluated, and to whom the results will be disclosed.
6. Determine and agree the appropriate method or combination of methods to be employed. Explain to, and gain the co-operation of, all participants.
7. Run the evaluation and analyse the results.
8. The steering group discusses the implications of the results and determines if change is necessary. The findings are shared as agreed in step five.
9. Formulate any required change and gain agreement from the stakeholders.
10. Implement the changes.

SUGGESTED FURTHER READING

Edwards, J. (1991) – Evaluation in Adult and Further Education. W.E.A. Liverpool

Gronlund, N.E. & Linn, R.L. (1990) – Measurement and Evaluation in Teaching. MacMillan Publishing Company, New York

Irby, D.M. (1983) – Evaluating Instruction in Medical Education: Journal of Medical Education 58, 844-49

Murphy, R. & Torrance, H. (1988) – Evaluating Education: Issues and Methods. Open University Press, Milton Keynes

Rowntree, D. (1981) – Developing Courses for Students. PCP Limited, London

Stenhouse, L. (1975) – An Introduction to Curriculum Research and Development. Heinmann, London

CHAPTER 8
The Educational Supervisor's Role in Medicine

COLIN COLES

INTRODUCTION

PERHAPS THE MOST crucial figure in ensuring the effectiveness of postgraduate medical training is the educational supervisor. Usually, the trainees' current consultant, it is the supervisor's task to ensure the trainee's educational needs are met. Until now, the educational supervisor's role has not been clearly described, nor have his or her tasks formed part of employment contracts or job plans.

This chapter addresses these issues by highlighting ten key elements essential in a good supervisor. These are equally applicable at the level of undergraduate and postgraduate education. The differences between assessment and appraisal are discussed, and the chapter concludes by discussing those issues that interfere with the development of sound educational supervision.

THE TEN ELEMENTS

Undoubtedly, being a successful educational supervisor takes time and effort. The job should not be grafted on to the work of an already over-stretched consultant. The role's full breadth must be clearly understood and acknowledged, since time and resources are necessary if educational supervision is to be efficient and effective.

Ten key elements are set out below. These constitute the basis of a job description for those who supervise medical staff training. This chapter will concentrate on discussing in some detail the essential ingredients of each element:

1. Be a good employer.
2. Be a mentor.
3. Create and maintain a conducive educational environment.
4. Provide opportunistic education.
5. Provide regular supervision.
6. Provide planned reviews of progress.
7. Contribute to formal education.
8. Offer counselling.
9. Conduct assessment of the trainee and the training provided.
10. Continue to be educated as an educator.

GOOD EMPLOYER

Above all, an educational supervisor should be a good employer. This means liaison with hospital management and contacting human resource or personnel departments about employment issues. It also involves communication with specialists and departmental colleagues concerning a particular post's educational provision and with clinical tutors regarding other more general educational issues.

First, the educational supervisor should ensure that there is a full and accurate job description for each training post. Such a description should include clear details of the nature, range and scope of the service work the trainee will be expected to undertake. It should also include the amount of clinical supervision available and should specify people (from various professions) who will be able to provide it. The job description should clearly state the post's educational opportunities and the educational supervision level, as distinct from clinical supervision. Finally, it should name the trainee's educational supervisor and other clinical teachers, and indicate when and how educational supervision will be provided.

The appointment process should be conducted according to good employment practice. This includes making available further particulars for the post, meeting applicants to discuss it prior to interview, and conducting the process itself appropriately. Interviewers should receive appropriate interview training.

In addition, trainees should be introduced to the trust, hospital, unit, and educational supervisor. This should be seen as a process spread over a period of time not something slotted into an already rushed and crowded first day. It should be planned in consultation with the clinical tutor and the human resources, or personnel, department.

Many hospital trusts today are part of the UK 'Investors in People' initiative. The national standards have implications for the education provided within a trust.

Investors in People: The National Standards

An investor in people:

- Makes a public commitment from the top down to develop all employees to achieve their objectives.
- Regularly reviews the training and development needs of all employees.
- Takes action to train and develop individuals on recruitment and through out their employment.
- Evaluates the investment in training and development to assess achievement and improve future effectiveness.

MENTOR

An educational supervisor should provide a good trainee role model. They learn a great deal through observation when no formal teaching is occurring. A trainee picks up informally what it is to be a good doctor. He or she does this by noting what senior colleagues, especially their supervisors, say and do. As far as trainees are concerned, the educational supervisor is constantly in the spotlight.

Being a mentor has two major components. He or she must be technically competent (and maintain that competence) and model appropriate attitudes that they communicate to trainees.

Secondly, a mentor should be open. Openness means being explicit about what one is doing, how one is doing it, and perhaps most importantly, why. The supervisor's actions should not be left for the trainee to interpret through guesswork. Openness also means being open to comment and criticism about one's professional actions. Supervisors should expect, and even encourage, trainees to have opinions and prepare them to discuss, not defend, their actions. Mentors should be confident in their professional relationship with their trainees in terms of both service and educational work. Striking a balance between these two is not easy, but the attempt indicates to trainees, a supervisor's commitment to their development.

CONDUCIVE EDUCATIONAL ENVIRONMENT

The educational supervisor's most important function is to establish and maintain an environment conducive to learning. It has three components:

First, the working environment should be one of honesty, trust, and fairness. People within a unit should be able to voice their thoughts without fear of repercussions. There should be a 'no blame' culture. There are two elements to this. First, celebrate everyone's successes and recognize that things go wrong because of the system and not because of any individual's poor practice. In short, there should be no 'scapegoating'. Second, supervisors should unconditionally support learners. It is all too easy for teachers at any level to forget or minimize what it was like not to know what they now know, or to be unable to do what they now do routinely. 'Unlearning' is difficult, but necessary. Supervisors must put themselves in the learner's position and unreservedly support and help them learn what might seem painfully obvious.

Third, the educational environment needs to be one where a spirit of inquiry – an evaluative culture – is constantly engendered. This can be achieved in numerous ways. Critique must be constructive and identify strengths as well as weaknesses. Next, learners need feedback on their performance successes, not only their failures. This is dealt with elsewhere, notably in Chapter Thirteen on Education in the Outpatient Clinic. Learners should monitor their own performance and engage in self-analysis leading to appropriate corrective action. After all, consultants moderate and adjust their own performance in relation to good practice criteria they established for themselves. Trainees learn this from their educational supervisors.

OPPORTUNISTIC EDUCATION:

The most significant educational opportunities occur in trainees' everyday work and during routine contact with their educational supervisors. For this reason alone, educational supervisors must have regular contact with trainees and their work. As often as possible, trainees should be observed at work. This also implies trainees watching their supervisors work.

Education may be particularly powerful during chance experiences that can have important learning outcomes. Therefore, through everyday contact, supervisors can contribute to establishing and maintaining the educational environment.

This does not mean that educational supervisors should be prepared to lecture on some particular topic at the drop of a hat. Rather, they should encourage trainees to see learning opportunities in everything they do. This also is explored elsewhere in this book.

REGULAR SUPERVISION

Educational supervisors should work with trainees regularly. Some of this supervision should involve the trainees' clinical practice, which is often neglected. Routine work provides numerous opportunities for learning. Trainees encounter new situations constantly. If they did not, they would not be trainees! The way they learn to perform new procedures and carry out novel tasks, and the way these are taught says a great deal about their training unit's educational quality. Put another way, to ensure trainees learn new clinical tasks, educational supervisors must put in place an appropriate system, or set of procedures. Sadly, this is often left to chance. Establish clear procedures if this responsibility is to be delegated to staff, such as other medical trainees or nurses. Such procedures might include identifying those accountable for this training, for record keeping of training, and for adequately training these trainers.

Educational supervision must be regular. Supervisors and trainees should meet both at work and away from it as often as possible in order to supervise thoroughly the trainee's educational progress. The frequency of these meetings should be determined by the clinical work and the educational supervisor's and trainee's job plans. The Royal College of Psychiatrists, in its 'trainee's charter', suggests regular supervision of one hour per week. To achieve regular supervision at anywhere near such a high level is certainly a challenge to other specialities. Whatever the frequency, trainees should be aware of how supervision is to be conducted within the unit in which they are working.

Regular educational supervision looks at both the trainees' current service provision and the unit clinicians' workload. It is a prime and early opportunity for educational supervisors to identify learning opportunities that trainees may undertake through self directed study. It is also a chance to give the trainee feedback. (See Chapter Two.) and contributes to the environment conducive to education described earlier. It helps to detect as early as possible and make the necessary provision for any problems that a trainee might encounter. Trainees also need opportunities to discuss career possibilities. This too can be addressed through regular supervision.

PLANNED PROGRESS REVIEWS

Educational supervisors should also give trainees planned progress reviews. Sometimes called 'appraisals', they offer opportunities of stepping back from daily education and service work and considering trainees' progress through the post and in their educational programme.

It is very important to begin progress reviews right at the start of a post, preferably within the first week. At this point, the supervisor finds out about the trainees' experience, hopes and expectations for this particular post. It is also an opportunity for trainees to discuss their career ideas in general. A trainee's ambitions for a career in general practice may determine what he or she will get out of the medical sub-speciality post they have been assigned to work in. Equally, the consultant must recognize that teaching trainees everything there is to know about the speciality is likely to be wasted effort if their ambitions lie elsewhere. This early meeting can discuss the post's educational opportunities, the kinds of clinical experience available, and the level of supervision provided. Much of this information will be available in printed form through the job description and could be reviewed at this first meeting.

The outcome of the discussions should be that the educational supervisor and trainee establish an educational plan for the post. It is important that the plan is negotiated. What the trainee *wants* to learn might not agree with what the educational supervisor believes the trainee *needs* to learn. It may be necessary for trade off on both sides. The educational plan should be agreed right at the start and should be written down for the benefit of both.

The importance of recording the educational plan becomes clear when, in perhaps two months time, trainee and supervisor review progress during a further appraisal meeting. Note achievements and discuss areas where the plan has not been addressed satisfactorily. Consider reasons for successes and failures, as well as contributory features within the training post including the level of educational supervision. Discuss them openly. As a result of this review, plan the remainder of the post in a spirit of negotiation. Identify achievable targets, and add time scales. Agree a date for the next progress review in a further two months time.

Reviews of progress can then proceed for the remainder of the post on the basis of this review/plan, review/plan.

FORMAL EDUCATION

The educational supervisor further provides formal education for trainees. Most likely this occurs at fixed times and within a predetermined programme. Many posts allow trainees the opportunity to attend a core educational programme together with other trainees. This enables them to practice effectively at the appropriate level in their post or to prepare for post-graduate examinations.

Formal education need not be rigid and regimented with lectures the only method used. Nor should these programmes' content reflect only the teachers' demands. Providing learner centred education through formal teaching is possible, although approaches adopted might be unfamiliar to some medical teachers.

Core educational programmes, as far as possible should relate to the trainee's everyday experiences. Linking formal teaching to clinical examples helps establish the relevance of what is being taught and learnt. Trainees should be encouraged in the best use of formal educational opportunities, and to 'capture the learning' perhaps through establishing and maintaining their own learning portfolio.

COUNSELLING

Educational supervisors should be able to counsel trainees in career and personal areas.

Understandably, career development will concern trainees. Post-graduate education often general in the early stages, leads to ever-greater specialisation. However, early in their careers trainees must decide what training to pursue.

Trainees must have the opportunity for confidential talks to their educational supervisor, about hopes, aspirations, doubts and fears. Trainees recognise medicine is changing rapidly. Some may fear that over-specialisation now might make them less flexible in this changing profession. These concerns might make trainees reluctant to commit themselves to particular career pathways. Sensitivity on the part of the supervisor is essential to enable trainees to 'open up' in these discussions.

The trainee's personal development is the second area where counselling may be necessary. It is important to note that personal counselling between trainee and educational supervisor should look solely at the impact of the individual's personal development on their work and education. Great sensitivity is required here, and educational supervisors with their breadth of experience and wisdom are able to provide a valuable resource. Again, it is important to have already established an environment conducive to education to provide for such sensitive discussions.

Counselling may seem outside their competence to some educational supervisors. It is important that those people recognise that counselling occurs at different levels. Basic counselling involves 'active listening', meaning asking open rather than closed questions, and allowing trainees to speak their minds. Acquiring these skills is relatively easy and many employers offer short seminars or workshops on basic techniques. Suitable programmes are offered for consultants interested in undertaking training at a more advanced level. Consultants should know enough about counselling, and counselling provision locally, to be of help to trainees. They should also know when and how to refer a trainee to someone more experienced when they feel unable to proceed further.

ASSESSMENT

Educational Supervisors are responsible for assessing both trainees and their training. It is important to recognise that the primary purpose of assessment is regulation. Its function is accreditation of both trainee, and training.

First consider trainee assessment. Educational supervisors must examine their trainees' clinical competence. Probably, these assessments will be for regulatory purposes, and unlike the progress reviews or appraisals mentioned above, will not be confidential. In the United Kingdom, the recent introduction of the Specialist Registrar raises the issue of how speciality colleges will assess trainees' clinical competence. At the time of writing this book, proposals and schemes have yet to be fully clarified.

It is worth noting here that there is a conflict of interest in the role of educational supervisor. Supervisors' assessment of clinical competence for regulatory purposes changes their role as trainee mentor and 'critical friend' to one of candidate and examiner. This dilemma facing all teachers and educators is one educational supervisors must resolve. Being clear and explicit to trainees about the assessment criteria being used, as opposed to merely appraising, can only help resolve this dilemma. (See below for the differences between appraisal and assessment).

Differences between Appraisal and Assessment		
	ASSESSMENT	APPRAISAL
Prime purpose	Career regulation	Educational
Participants	Assessors and trainee	Appraiser and trainee (normally 1 to 1)
Methods	Variety	Appraisal interview
Areas covered	Generic skills e.g. communication Clinical skills and competence Management skills	Educational, personal and professional development Career progress Employment issues
Main activity	College assessments College examinations	Appraisal discussions
Informed by	Local assessment ratings	Trainee's self-assessment Day-to-day observation by trainers Other work-related inputs Results of assessments and examinations
Standards of achievement applied	External	Internal (personal to the trainee) and negotiated with the appraiser
Output documentation	Certificate of passing assessments and examinations Feedback on performance in assessments	Record of appraisal having taken place Agreed educational and personal development plan
Disclosure	Yes	No (see discussion)
Review/appeal	College exams - mostly no Local assessments - yes	No (decisions should always be joint ones)
Outcome	Career progression	Enhanced educational, personal and professional development

Second, training assessment focuses primarily on the post, the educational qualities of the supervisor and other teachers and the training system in which they all operate. There should be a mechanism for monitoring what training is provided and when, how both trainees and trainers perceive its quality, together with records of educational outcomes.

Clearly, this is new territory for many educational supervisors who have little experience of assessing the quality of the training being provided. In some settings, clinical tutors use trainee questionnaires to monitor training provision and quality. This information can be fed back to supervisors and others responsible for training posts in order to develop posts to even higher standards of educational provision.

With the introduction of educational contracts between post-graduate deans and hospital trusts for the provision of high quality training, it is likely that this monitoring of educational provision could be used for regulatory purposes and for training-post accreditation. Currently, visits by speciality college panels can lead to the withdrawal of training approval. Post-graduate deans might well develop similar mechanisms to support their educational contracts.

Educational supervisors and other educators associated with postgraduate education should develop criteria for assessing their educational provision. The ten roles of the educational supervisor being described here might form a basis for this.

An important consideration in establishing criteria for educational provision monitoring is the relationship between education provided and clinical service to patients. This harks back to the earlier discussion of the potential conflict between education and service work. It would be useful for educational supervisors, together with their colleagues within units and departments, to monitor their educational provision, in part to clarify their educational activity.

Then, in discussion with colleagues and managers, educational activity could feature more significantly than at present in consultants' job plans. Equally, there must be discussions with the purchasers of health care to ensure that education and training are as much part of the 'contract price' as the more direct costs of providing clinical services.

EDUCATING THE EDUCATORS

The educational supervisor's final role is to ensure that he or she understands and puts into practice the principles underpinning education. In short, supervisors must develop their skills as educators.

Until now, educational supervision has been largely an amateur pursuit. There was some provision of education for educators at local and regional level both across and within specialities. Some clinicians sufficiently self-motivated to pursue their studies in education have undertaken higher degrees in the subject. A growing number of masters programmes in medical education are currently offered, mostly on a part-time and distance learning basis to suit consultants' busy work schedules. A small number of clinicians are undertaking research degrees such as (MPhil and PhDs) in education.

Programmes, such as Advanced Trauma Life Support, already demand that trainers undergo formal instruction in course delivery to ensure maximum learning for trainees. These requirements may become more commonplace. Meanwhile, the quality of *educating the educators programmes* needs further development. Indeed, more evaluation of the effects of these programmes on instructors' educational performance is required. Limited research has currently been undertaken in this field, and those studies that do exist suggest educating the educators, provided it is conducted appropriately, can enhance learning.

BARRIERS TO DEVELOPING EDUCATIONAL SUPERVISION

While describing these ten features of an educational supervisor's role, it is recognised that a number of barriers limit development. These barriers must be acknowledged, discussed, and addressed. Many of these are deeply embedded and reflect traditional assumptions within medicine itself.

There is a changing ethos within medicine. Trainees today, along with some specialist staff too, see medicine less as a profession and more as a job of work. In recent years, the debate over junior doctors' hours and working conditions has contributed to this change. When asked to attend early morning educational sessions before service work some trainees demand an earlier close to the day. This 'clock watching' is an anathema to some supervisors and can lead to a less than positive trainer/trainee relationship.

Previously, education was often haphazard and opportunistic. People learned largely on-the-job. Indeed, a junior doctor's time was mostly spent in caring for patients. Now, most trainees are in post to become fully qualified as quickly as possible. This is not to say that trainees cannot learn very effectively through their service work. Indeed, chapters in this book indicate effective and efficient ways this can happen. Nevertheless, in this new era, the trainees are there to learn and not simply to do the work. Again, some supervisors have difficulty adjusting to this notion.

Today, there is a new educational philosophy in place and it forms a further barrier to educational supervision. The emphasis is on understanding learning and learner rather than teacher and teaching concerns. Indeed, as is being described throughout this book, teaching is the facilitation of learning. Any educational experience should be seen from the learner's point of view. If one understands what learning means, then one knows how to teach it. Approach to education is more learner-centred. This has not been part of many consultants' experience in their own education, and some find it difficult to adopt.

There have also been social changes. While previously, there were clear work relationship hierarchies with 'bosses' in authority over other members of staff, now there is a greater sense of workplace equality. At all staffing levels more and more people are on first name terms. Whatever differences there might be in status or salary, there is a greater sense of equality than before. Again, this is not always something that has formed the experience of those consultants who are now educational supervisors. Many may find these changes uncomfortable. They expect people to 'do as they say' without contradiction. Open discussion on issues becomes difficult.

Another barrier to developing educational supervision is that education is contracted out. As already mentioned, post-graduate deans hold hospital unit educational contracts for providing education for doctors in training. These contracts allow a proportion of trainees' salary costs to be held by the post-graduate dean. If satisfactory education and training is not provided in accordance with the educational contract, post-graduate deans can withdraw this funding. Good education is now a contractual obligation.

Finally, *patronage* is a concern. Trainees may feel obligated to their consultant since, at the end of the post, he or she must sign up the trainee to indicate satisfactory completion of the post. Moreover, trainees might have ambitions to secure a further post with the same consultant or with the consultant's colleagues. This knowledge might well restrict the level of openness and honesty the trainee feels able to give in his or her relationship with the educational supervisor. This is a strong reason for the emphasis of this chapter on the importance of consultants establishing and maintaining a positive and conducive educational environment.

CONCLUSION

The educational supervisor is crucial to the provision of education in the workplace. In the past, the role has not been clearly specified but seen as an intrusive part of any consultant's workload. With very little in the way of formal training, there was a consequent wide variety in terms of the extent and quality of the supervision.

This chapter sets out in detail ten elements that must be addressed for success in the role. Some of the barriers to implementation are discussed along with ways of overcoming them. Success as a supervisor requires an interest in developing the role and the dedication of time and effort to fulfill it. Management and colleagues in their turn must acknowledge those efforts. Time and resources need to be allocated. Part of the driving force will be the contracting process and the post-graduate deans' consequent allocation of funds.

SUGGESTED FURTHER READING

Bond, D. (1995) – Enhancing Learning through Self-Assessment. Kogan Page, London

Coles, C. & Holm, H.A. (1993) – Learning in Medicine. Scandinavian University Press

Fish, D. & Coles, C. (1973) – Developing Professional Judgement in Healthcare. Learning the critical appreciation of practice. Butterworth Heinemann, London

Fish, D. & Twinn, S. (1997) – Quality Clinical Supervision in the Health Care Professions; Principled Approaches to Practice. Butterworth Heinemann, London

THE PRACTICE

'... Theory without practice is sterile'

Chapters nine to fourteen consider teaching and learning in the clinical setting, either in hospital or general practice. Each has its own particular strengths and weaknesses and teachers have their own individual styles. Based on the preceding chapters, various teaching situations are discussed with a view to making the best use of the teaching opportunities presenting themselves daily.

Small group work is particularly highlighted in chapters nine to eleven, whether in the journal club context or on the wards. Chapter twelve discusses the teaching of practical skills, particularly in the theatre environment. Such techniques are readily transferable to the teaching of any skill a doctor has to undertake, from using an ophthalmoscope to the insertion of a chest drain. Teaching in outpatient clinics or in general practice is covered in chapter thirteen and finally, chapter fourteen is devoted to the preparation and delivery of lectures.

CHAPTER 9
Journal Clubs & Critical Reading

RODNEY PEYTON

INTRODUCTION

JOURNAL CLUBS have existed in some form for over a century. During that time the numbers of papers and communications increased exponentially. In any major subject, tens of thousands of research papers are produced annually. This is enough to swamp even the most die-hard reader. However, they do represent the leading edge of medical progress, either as original articles or overviews.

By their very nature, textbooks lag at least five years behind. This is unfortunate since the current rapid change in all forms of knowledge requires an equally rapid educational and personal development process. All professionals must keep up to date in their subject. They can achieve this in a variety of ways.

Attending courses or lectures may help, but this can be expensive in terms of both time and money.

If used properly, journal clubs, represent one of the most cost-effective methods for the provision of continuing medical education.

Unfortunately, since many clinicians feel such meetings are non-productive, even boring, they are poorly attended. Commonly, meetings are disorganised, lack a clear aim and have little demonstrable relevance to clinical practice. Outside major centres limited direct or 'on line' library services can be restrictive.

This chapter aims to define a journal club's objectives, consider the ideal format, and suggest an approach to critical reading. It concludes with an overview of those features associated with a successful programme.

THE PURPOSE OF A JOURNAL CLUB

One of the most fundamental skills in any professional's *armamentarium* is the ability to reflect on current practice in the light of new information. In times of rapid change, this is not merely a useful skill but a professional responsibility. Such reflection must become a habit. Forming a group to aid in the process reinforces and supplements other self-learning techniques such as personal reading or attendance at lectures and talks.

Debating issues is vital training for those new to the profession. It does not just keep them up-dated but creates insight into developments. Such debate helps clarify and solidify opinions, thereby instilling the confidence to use new knowledge in clinical practice.

Most papers present research on the outcome of experimentation, clinical observation or retrospective analysis. The need to analyse such results led some to conclude that all practitioners must have research experience. However, many with busy schedules and short training cycles do not wish to devote time to research, a valid reason. However, in order to analyse others' research designs and results and weigh the evidence all must be familiar with the design process, protocols and ethics associated with research. This involves epidemiology and biostatistics studies best discovered and remembered in a clinical context although they can be learned separately. An understanding of experimental design and techniques leads to an understanding of the necessity for clear definition of research questions. Carried through to clinical practice this assists the auditing process essential for the reflective practitioner.

While the overriding purpose of journal clubs is evaluating research and disseminating information on good practice, there are two added benefits. Firstly, the use of small group discussion where everyone is free to express their opinion can enhance relationships within a unit. It also allows those in a supervisory role to assess and guide the development of professional ethics by actively listening to group members' contributions. This includes assessment of interpersonal skills and the ability to debate issues with other professionals.

Secondly, journal clubs are an opportunity for practising and improving presentation skills. The ability to stand up in front of a group to relate the salient points of a piece of research is a valuable asset. Properly managed, journal clubs provide not only a cost effective and efficient method of keeping up to date in clinical practice, but also a method for early development of particular skills trainees will need throughout their professional life. In order to benefit from the session, journal club facilitators must be experienced clinicians and teachers.

FORMAT

The sessions must be clearly focused and papers chosen for analysis should be as relevant as possible to the group's clinical needs. A one-hour session normally allows in-depth discussion of four papers at most.

There tend to be two basic formats. In the first, three or four members each prepare and present a paper. This is a prime micro-teaching technique (see Chapter Ten) with a five to seven minute presentation of relevant findings and a short critical analysis.

The rest of the group can focus on discussing the paper or a clinical situation. This is, probably, the most efficient use of preparation time.

However, another widely used technique calls for the facilitator to select and issue a number of papers to all group members two days in advance so that everyone may read them and form their own conclusions. This is best if there is relevant clinical material on which to base conclusions for future practice. After this, the facilitator chairs an open discussion. It is rarely necessary for discussions in either format to last more than fifteen or twenty minutes. The chairperson or facilitator guides the discussion, encouraging all members. The aim is to reach some form of conclusion with clinical practice implications and, where appropriate, formulate a plan of action to achieve the change.

Clearly, the whole process depends on participants being well grounded in critical reading skills. These must be developed at an early stage of a professional's career and can be helped by a handout that serves as an *aide memoire* to the critique. The next section covers this in more detail.

CRITICAL READING

Most papers in journals fall into one of two categories, either original research or review articles/editorials. These will be considered in turn.

Research Papers

Since the importance of research in advancing clinical practice is beyond dispute, junior staff are expected to develop research skills and produce papers during their training. Unfortunately, a significant number undertake such investigations simply to be able to fill that box in the curriculum vitae entitled 'Research'. Similar pressures force institutions to justify research grants by publishing constantly. Consequently, there is a plethora of publications and, in order to determine the relevance of the research findings to his or her clinical practice, readers of even the most eminent must develop analytical skills.

SELECTION OF PAPERS

With the proliferation of research papers, comes an increase in the number of journals available. Although, one of the lesser-known journals may contain some pertinent work, the odds are very much against it. Authors want to enhance their reputations by giving their work the widest and most weighty exposure. It is best to be selective and read three or four reputable journals in a particular subject area.

Having identified the appropriate journals, scan the list of contents and pick out relevant titles. Only when the summary is read should a decision be made as to whether or not the article is worth reading in detail. If the summary indicates no relationship to clinical practice, the paper should be discarded. Similarly, if the summary is not succinct and well written, the quality of the paper is probably suspect and should be rejected.

When reviewing a selected paper the reader must approach the task with purpose. The following provides a guide to the critical appraisal of each section.

Introduction

The most important element of the introduction is the statement of the research aim. This should be worded clearly. It is worthwhile remembering that, by the nature of things, the 'statement of research question' may be determined after the research has been completed! The paper itself may be an offshoot of a totally different intention. Careful scrutiny of the statement of aim reveals obvious bias. For instance, a statement such as 'the purpose of this study was to prove…' should alert the reader to a possible bias. Establish whether the paper is the result of an experiment, clinical observations, or a retrospective analysis.

134

The research problem should be stated clearly. The introduction should discuss possible significance for practice. Any literature cited should be directly relevant, not just to the topic, but to the question under consideration. By the end of the introduction the reader should understand why this particular research was undertaken and be able to determine the relevance of any findings to his or her own clinical practice. Note, however, setting the problem in a different context can make it more personally relevant than the author intended.

Materials and Methods

This section details the subject population and justifies research instrument selection.

—*Subjects:* Was an entire population studied and was it appropriate to the problem? If the population was large, was an appropriate sample selected and was the method used clearly described and justified? Were there any exclusions, and why? Did this method make obvious sense or was there any bias in selection, for example age, gender or race? This feature is sometimes glossed over and yet can invalidate the whole exercise. Therefore, time should be taken to look carefully at this particular aspect.

—*Instruments:* Check the measurement method used and whether it was appropriate. Was the sample size adequate for this particular technique? Does it, of itself, have any bias towards a particular part of the population, for instance, in language use? Who administered the instrument and was this appropriate? A single observer can introduce possible bias while many can result in different interpretations of the answers. What was the response rate and was it reasonable? Was the instrument reliable for a particular problem at a particular time and in a particular place? Was it necessary to have a control population and, if so, was this appropriately chosen and examined? The reader should always look to his or her own experience and determine other variables that could influence the outcome and note if these were included.

Results

This section should present the findings and their significance in as straightforward a manner as possible. Are the results described fully and clearly and are they likely to be reproducible? Which statistical tests were used and why? This clearly implies that the basics of biostatistics must be understood. This includes levels of significance and the difference between the use of parametric and non-parametric tests. What level of significance was achieved? Statements such as 'These results almost achieved statistical significance' should raise suspicion. This means they were not significant and should not be given undue credence. Further, it warns of possible bias. Before reading the author's conclusions, readers should make up their own minds about the significance of the results with respect to the question posed. Only then should the discussion section be read.

Discussion/Conclusions

This section should present argument consistent with the findings leading to a logical conclusion and recommendations for practice. It should not rehash the results section. Discussion of each result should relate to the original problem. Before reaching a conclusion as to clinical significance, each finding should be compared with other literature that considers both sides of the argument. When research is carried out under specific conditions, conclusions should not be generalised to the whole population without convincing arguments. In other words, be alert for authors arguing from the particular to the general or vice versa. Would the same conclusion be valid under different circumstances? For instance, would there be other variables not examined in the present research?

If the paper's findings appear valid for a particular research study, consideration should be given to their implications for clinical practice both in terms of feasibility and from a moral or ethical standpoint. In particular, are these findings sufficiently robust to entertain a change in practice and if so, is this to be on a long term or on an experimental basis?

Review Articles and Editorials

The other main publications in journals are reviews of recent research findings, either as articles or editorial comment presenting a more personal perspective. When well written these save time spent reading research papers in many journals. However, the articles do have to be evaluated critically. Comments in the most reputable journals should be read carefully since reviewers are likely to be biased.

Note the country or institution of origin and consider whether these are known to have any differences in clinical practice. Next, the introductory and concluding paragraphs should be read to see if they relate well to one another. Decide if the findings match expectations and common practice. If so, scan the article for any new information and, if none is apparent, take no further action.

Should conclusions prove new or suggest changes in practice, they should be followed closely and original articles obtained. This step cannot be overemphasised. It is negligent to change practice without such enquiry. Subject the articles to the same scrutiny as any other research paper (see above) before entertaining a change in clinical practice.

From the above, it is obvious there is a considerable amount of work involved in reading research papers and review articles. It is a clinician's duty to evaluate the information so that patient management is not altered on the basis of research findings that may not stand the test of time. The potential for critical debate in a journal club makes it an excellent forum to discuss the pros and cons of any new technique before its introduction into the clinical environment. How does one keep up the momentum of a journal club and ensure high attendance? The final section will look at those features known to help in this process.

135

RUNNING A SUCCESSFUL JOURNAL CLUB

Success is never accidental. It requires commitment, careful planning and sound organisation by those responsible for running the club.

Characteristics of a Successful Club
- Clear aim
- Clinically relevant
- Routine meetings approximately once per month
- Experienced facilitator
- Small groups with similar clinical interests
- High expectation of attendance–led by example
- Critical appraisal skills taught at an early stage
- Freedom to debate openly and express opinions
- All members involved in decision making
- Summary produced with plan for action.

136

Successful clubs achieve their aim, attract membership and are influential in improving practice. Typically, they are guided by a small number of motivated and skilled facilitators who help select topics directly relevant to the group in its everyday clinical activity. There must be a clear aim. The group should agree on structure and direction to give everyone a sense of ownership. Opinions must be freely and openly expressed and debated. This can be a problem if there is a wide range of seniority.

A clear routine is very important. Groups should meet at an appropriate venue once a month on a set day and at a time mutually convenient. Even if it is not absolutely mandatory, attendance should be expected. Organisation ensuring disturbance by neither bleep nor telephone is required. Usually, it is possible to arrange for emergencies arising during the session to be dealt with by one designated team member.

Small groups from one unit or others in a similar field are usually best at keeping the topics focused. Critical reading skills should be taught at an early stage, perhaps with a refresher at the beginning of each academic year. The facilitator's role becomes crucial in maintaining the standard of debate, as he or she guides and protects group members to encourage participation.

Finally, as with any other educational experience, adult education principles should obtain the maximum benefit. (See Chapter Two). Successful clubs have well-motivated participants who feel the sessions are relevant. They are given time to reflect on how the information presented relates to everyday clinical practice. The summary that, if relevant, should include a plan of action providing feedback after the group discussion. Clinical audit should be the process the group uses to review outcomes of any changes in practice.

CONCLUSION

In this information age, it is estimated the knowledge base in medicine doubles every two to three years. New ideas are generated and old ones discarded. Clinicians must keep abreast of the cutting edge in their speciality in order to maintain their professional credibility. The reading of journals must become a habit from a very early stage in a professional career. The knowledge gained must be fully evaluated before being clinical use. Critical debate with others in a similar field best achieves this. This allows for confidence when new ideas are put into action.

Therefore, journal clubs provide a very important method of continuing medical education for the reflective practitioner. It should be seen not as an obligation but as a gateway to success in professional practice.

CHAPTER 10
Small Group Teaching in the Medical Context

139

MIKE WALKER

INTRODUCTION

THOSE WHO CHOOSE to write about teaching and learning in small groups, more often than not, do so from a committed position. They both describe and advocate it. Beginning with the supposed ills of alternative methods, principally the lecture and the seminar, they present the former as a highly didactic event restricting the audience to passive information and fact gathering. In the seminar, a student presents a paper that the group, led by the tutor, demolishes.

These negative caricatures are not altogether accurate although there are easily recognisable elements. In fact, most of us can recall the occasional brilliant lecture, inspirational seminar or revelatory small group discussion. In truth, these valued educational episodes tend to be few, not through any one method's merits or demerits, but because of the teacher's competence or lack of it. One can advocate teaching methods and list their advantages, but it is the teacher's knowledge, skill and enthusiasm that matters. This chapter not only describes small group teaching methods but also should help readers develop their personal competence as teachers.

WHY SMALL GROUPS?

Small group teaching is seen as appropriate for any set of learners from primary school onwards. However, it seems particularly appropriate for adults. Unlike children or undergraduate students, adults bring to their learning a clear sense of purpose. Adults usually engage in learning in order to achieve some end that is important to them as individuals. This will often be concerned with their day-to-day work, with longer term career aspirations, with professional goals or with some non-professional ambition, (to play a musical instrument, restore a vintage car or learn Spanish). Adults decide to learn because they have a specific need or purpose for that learning. They will be motivated to the extent that their educational experience is meaningful and relevant in pursuing their purpose.

There are a number of ideas that resonate with small group teaching. To begin with small group methods not only convey information but help learners understand that information. Through discussion, small groups foster intellectual skills such as reasoning, evaluating, making judgements, applying principles. As well, they learn social skills such as listening, responding, collaborating and so on. Small groups require participation and are an active means of learning. They encourage self-expression and the building of a coherent personal philosophy. Although, we do not expect to have to articulate all our views on jobs, careers, life and everything else, we all have them. In the current climate of accountability, young professionals, Pre-Registration House Officers and Senior House Officers, for instance, may be required to give account of themselves and their actions. Of course, junior doctors have their personal understanding and rationalisations, but personal understanding remains just that - personal - unless we can test our ideas against others. Personal understanding requires public validation.

Through small groups it is possible to turn personal understanding into a coherent, rational and professionally defensible position that can be confidently articulated. Arguably, senior doctors having such skills already would find less value in small group discussion. However, there are two reasons why this is not the case. The first is that when asked if they learn most through lectures, personal study, conferences, seminars, audit meetings and so on, invariably doctors shake their heads and say they learn most from discussion with colleagues. The benefit of such naturally occurring learning methods should be brought into the educational context and exploited. The second reason for believing consultants might benefit from small group discussion concerns the current upsurge of interest in medical education. Doctors tend to have little, if any, formal training in education. If they are interested in education and becoming skilled teachers, then there is a universe of discourse they must explore and small group discussion seems to be most appropriate for this exploration.

TYPES OF SMALL GROUPS AND THEIR USES

Up to twenty-eight ways of working with small groups have been identified. Within the context of postgraduate medical education perhaps five are really relevant:

1. Seminar
2. Closed discussion
3. Open discussion
4. Workshops
5. Groups without tutor.

SEMINAR

Teaching and learning though seminars may be the most familiar form of group work and is widely used in both hospital departments and postgraduate centres. In universities, it is based upon presenting a paper or reading an essay followed by comment and criticism. In its medical form, the seminar is based upon presenting and debating a case. This author's recent research on the training of junior hospital doctors describes a weekly departmental seminar in a London teaching hospital in the following way.

> The room is rather cramped. The chairs are set out in rows facing the front. The front row is occupied by four consultants (in suits). In the second and third rows are two registrars and two senior registrars (in sports jackets) and in the remaining rows, wearing white coats, are four senior house officers (SHO).
>
> Dr. Woods (SHO) is asked to begin the presentation. He spends 3 - 4 minutes sorting X-ray plates and putting them on the screen. The others chat. Dr. Woods asks if there is an OHP. Mr. Richardson (consultant) puts the data up on the TV screen for him, but it's too small, so he has to read it out. He goes over to the X-ray plates to illustrate a point, but seems unable to make any sense of what he sees. Mr. Olsen gets up and re-orders the plates, turns some around and some the other way up. He then gives a lucid explanation of what the plates show. Mr. Moffat questions one of his statements. They go into discussion, joined by Mr. Scott. Dr. Woods sits on one side and takes no more part in the proceedings. Two of the other SHOs have left to answer bleep calls. The fourth says nothing.

While the consultants here may be learning a great deal from collegiate discussion, it is difficult to see what Dr. Woods or the other SHOs present might have got from this exercise. Whatever the seminar's merits, the SHOs in this version were not being enabled to explore, develop and articulate ideas. This is not to suggest that the seminar as a means of teaching and learning be at fault, only that in this particular example SHO learning was not promoted.

It also raises fundamental medical education issues in hospitals. This seminar contains all grades of hospital doctors on an ostensibly egalitarian, 'We are all equal as scholars' basis. At the same time, there are huge discrepancies in experience, knowledge, understanding and most important of all, needs. What the SHO needs to know is not what the consultant or the registrar need to know. Contributions to seminar debate will vary in the same way.

How might Dr. Woods and the other SHOs have contributed to the discussion between consultants? The level of debate was prohibitive, but there was another reason. In order to demonstrate competence to senior doctors, juniors must give a sound account of cases. They feel that they have to impress. Could the SHOs risk a contribution that was less than impressive? It would seem that the status distinction between junior doctors and consultants is a barrier to learning, particularly to SHO learning in the public forum of a seminar. How might matters be improved for Dr. Woods and his colleagues? First, here are some organisational suggestions. Afterwards, some more fundamental issues might need to be considered.

It is possible to present cases well, using properly prepared and imaginative techniques and involving more than one SHO. Thereafter, one of the consultants might have run a small discussion group with the SHOs while the other three joined the registrars for discussion. The two groups could have eventually joined and each reported their conclusions before continuing with a joint discussion, with summary and conclusions. However, if consultants relish their sometimes, adversarial debate in front of their juniors, then such a change in organisation would be resisted.

The seminar with case study can be useful for teaching and learning. The cases provide relevance to everyday work, issues and problems. Senior doctors act as models in terms of explanation, research and management. Indeed, identifying techniques for management may be the most obviously useful part of the seminar for SHOs. However, the discussion may also help them understand the case through reflection.

In their review of the training of junior hospital doctors, the Standing Committee on Postgraduate Medical Education (SCOPME) recognised the potential of hospital work as a source of experiential learning. They also recognised the necessity of reflection.

> Time to reflect and learn is clearly a key factor in any educational system and the learning environment must provide ample opportunity for this for both trainers and trainees.

The seminar is usually somewhat larger than a small group discussion. For this chapter's purposes it will be defined as being composed of one leader and three to five participants. There are four principal approaches, closed discussion, open discussion, workshop, and tutor-less group.

THE CLOSED DISCUSSION

The closed discussion is usually task-centred, with the group providing the task, problem or question. Since the discussion's purpose is resolving issues and achieving a consensus upon which policy decisions may be made, it follows that closed discussions will be used where there is a real possibility of achieving some unanimity. Possible topics for closed discussion might include:

- treatment of acute tonsillitis
- the use of chest drains in pneumonectomy
- the safe use of diathermy
- the management of a cardiac arrest.

The leader of the closed discussion canvases views, using closed questions, and noting replies. She or he keeps the group on task and offers summaries during and at the end of the discussion.

THE OPEN DISCUSSION

The open discussion is process- rather than task-centred. To the individual, its value lies in participation rather than in resolving group tasks, since individuals find open discussion topics the most relevant. These concern issues and dilemmas with no clear and unambiguous guidelines provided by medical science. Possible topics for open discussion might include.

- What constitutes informed consent?
- The significance of patient beliefs for GP Consultations.
- Cost and its influence on treatment.
- A request for contraceptive pills from a 13 year old girl.
- The value of learning contracts for SHOs.
- Breaking bad news.

The open discussion leader generally asks questions and attempts, through his or her responses, to encourage individuals to develop their ideas through discourse with the other members of the group. The aim is to help all group members to express their views and receive feedback from others. This requires the leader to have a range of skills which will be discussed later. At the end of the discussion, the leader summarises, perhaps in open discussion, all viewpoints expressed.

WORKSHOPS

Usually, workshops are associated with a practical skill station such as suturing or insertion of a chest drain. The discussion ensures that learners have understood the underlying issues, can recognise and interpret patterns. It is concerned with the cognitive or conceptual elements of the skill, and offers an opportunity to fix the skill verbally. As well, it helps learners understand the principles behind its use. The leader needs to establish the learners' existing knowledge base and continually relate to it through questions and answers. Discussion is interspersed with periods of skills practice. The session should close with the leader establishing what has been learned by each member and then providing a summary.

TUTOR-LESS GROUPS

Tutor-less groups are often used to break up a larger or more formal presentation. The large group is split into smaller groups of three to five members who are given a task to complete within a specified time. Whatever the task - to devise a means of assessing skill stations, to identify objectives for a course on consultation skills, to develop strategies for teaching rhythm recognition - it should be specific. It is important to check that the group members understand the task. Usually, discussion gets under way fairly quickly. If it does not there may be a problem with the task or its appropriateness. Initially, 15 minutes is allowed for the exercise although it could stretch to 30 minutes if it proves to be particularly useful. During this time the organiser would move between groups, listening and checking that the group is functioning, is on task, on time and still productive. At 'time' the groups report on their deliberations via a single spokesperson, often assisted by an OHP acetate the group prepares. The work of each small group will be commented on and perhaps discussed by the remainder of the large group.

Tutor-less groups allow for active and relevant involvement in the midst of a more formal and passive session. They allow for collegial discussion and feedback and may also produce some genuine solutions to collective problems. But they may do more than this. From the organiser's point of view the difficult part begins with group presentations. The organiser's task is to discern within these presentations, trends, themes and commonalties, to identify these and to produce a synthesis of the ideas offered. For instance, if the groups are to identify the circumstances under which they learn best, then it is usually possible to produce from their responses a synthesis approximating adult learning principles. It is this synthesis that is most likely to result in the development of genuinely new insights for the learners. Whatever the outcome of the tutorless group discussion, it needs to be related to and incorporated within the reconvened whole group session. Tutor-less groups may, of course be used to begin or end a teaching session although they are seldom used as the only teaching strategy.

OBJECTIVES

The course programme specifies that it is a 'Small group discussion' so it is really necessary to state objectives? After all, everyone knows how to discuss and we generally find it an enjoyable and sometimes worthwhile activity. If members get into small groups and chat for a while, then they must learn something. So is it really necessary to have objectives? Yes! If it is not possible to specify in advance what learning is expected then it is not possible to tell whether the objectives, or anything else, have been achieved. Secondly, discussion is the means or the method not the substance or content of what the participants learn. It is important to specify carefully what knowledge, skills or attitudes are to be acquired through the medium of discussion.

For discussion, two kinds of objective can be distinguished. Task objectives relate to the outcomes of the discussion. For instance, the group may be given the task of identifying appropriate methods for evaluating a course. Process objectives on the other hand are concerned with what the individual members should gain from the discussion. Thus, it is important to establish whether the task or the process objectives are to be the most important. For workshops, normally the task objectives predominate. Some examples of objectives follow:

Task Objectives
   By the end of the discussion group members will have:
   • Expressed their views in relation to safety in the operating theatre.
   • Produced an agreed list of safe practices.
   • Produced a list of suggestions for implementing these practices.
Process Objectives
   By the end of the discussion group members will have:
   • Explored a range of views on 'listening to the patient'.
   • Evaluated the view of others and reflected upon their own views.
   • Developed their personal understanding of the significance of 'listening to the patient'.
Workshop Objectives
   By the end of the workshop, group members will:
   • Know the principles of the closed and open methods of introducing pneumoperitoneum.

- Know and have practised a safe method for inserting a Verres needle.
- Understand the potential complications of pnuemoperitoneum.

The workshop differs from the skill station in its inclusion of a (usually closed) discussion of the principles underlying the use of the skill, its performance and the implications of its use.

PRE-DISCUSSION ACTIVITIES

Asking group members to undertake some activity prior to the group meeting may help maximise the achievement of objectives by the end of the discussion. For instance, they may be given the topic and asked to:

- Focus their thinking
- Collect personal examples and illustrations related to the topic
- Spend some time observing an area related to the topic and collect some original data
- Canvas the opinions of colleagues and patients.
- Read a handout or library material.

Any of these activities ensures a common base from which to begin. However, an informed guess of the number of participants likely to complete such pre-course activities would be prudent. If the realistic estimate is, 'few if any', then ascertaining the extent of their experience and knowledge may have to form part of the introduction, alongside name, place of work and so on. A further suggestion in such cases is to ask one member to work up a short, up to five minute, presentation in advance of the meeting. This would include a so-called micro-teaching episode, that is, a review of basic topic-related principles and concepts so that participants have a reasonable basis for the session. In the light of information gathered at the start of the session, the leader's adopted role may need adjustment.

LEADERSHIP ROLES

It will be apparent that each of the three types of group discussion briefly described requires different behaviour from the group leader. This section outlines some of the possible roles or modes group leaders may adopt.

CHAIRPERSON

Probably, this is the most familiar role. The chairperson initiates and controls proceedings seated prominently, perhaps at the head of the table. The 'chair' is highly task-centred and keeps the group on task, remains neutral in terms of content and may show concern for correct procedures. The chairperson's role fits more readily with a closed discussion.

FACILITATOR

The facilitator sits within the circle and is indistinguishable from group members. She or he asks minimal, open questions or responds in other ways only when the discussion appears to be unproductive. The facilitator is highly process-centred and sensitive to relationships and their part in enhancing individual understanding within the group. The facilitator role is best suited to open discussion.

INSTRUCTOR

The instructor occupies a prominent position at, or seated near, a skill station. She or he initiates and organises demonstrations, discussions and skill practices. Usually, the discussion is closed with the instructor as chairperson. The discussion will be task-centred and focus upon both the principles behind the skill and its performance. However, since an adequate grasp of either needs to relate to previous experience, the instructor may need, at some points, to move into a more open discussion. The instructor role is clearly best suited to workshops.

146

PARTICIPANT

Operating as a group participant has its attractions. Leading a group is hard work whereas participation is usually enjoyable and rewarding without responsibility. However, discussion without a leader is a rudderless ship. It is difficult to imagine achieving certain objectives in a group without a leader. Simple participation is not recommended.

DEVIL'S ADVOCATE

Probably, the devil's advocate has been involved in many similar courses in the past and may have led many group discussions on this or related topics. She or he knows all the arguments and switches eloquently from one to another without apparent contradiction. Whatever is said the devil's advocate knows the perfect counter-argument. The problem is that this person's responses are often driven by a personal need to demonstrate knowledge, skill, and wit rather than by the needs of the group.

AGITATOR

The agitator dislikes comfortable discussion, believing it intellectual game-playing. This person believes that only stirring the emotions makes for meaningful personal statements. The agitator probes and retorts to invoke anger, aggression, fear, and indignation, all for group exploration.

No doubt, there are many more variations upon the role of group leader. However, it is difficult to see a place for either devil's advocate or agitator within an educational enterprise. Whatever role is adopted must always include certain basics. The leader must communicate the discussion's purpose and introduce the objectives, as well as, ensure that group members understand what has to be done. As he or she is responsible for ensuring that objectives are achieved, this usually requires some mental withdrawal from the debate in order to check progress. Also, it requires checking and ensuring that there is enough time for the closure process.

ENVIRONMENT

In our ordinary day-to-day activities we take some care over the environments we inhabit. Our homes are arranged to fit with the kinds of lives we lead and if we decide to have a house or dinner party we may go to some lengths to arrange rooms and furniture so as to be conducive to our purpose. Whether in theatre or a GP surgery, the environment: lighting, heating, the stationing of furniture and people, must all be appropriate to the task. If one element is out of place, say it is too cold or ventilation is poor, then the performance of tasks may be impaired. So it is with discussions. If they are to work at their best, and indeed, if they are to work at all, the environment has to be right.

Imagine a room 30 yards long and 15 yards wide. The ceiling is twice as high as a normal room. There are no windows, but fluorescent strips light up the dull green picture-less walls. In the middle of the room, on the vinyl flooring stand eight metal chairs arranged for discussion. This is not exactly a conducive environment for discussion. Imagine a second room, once the drawing room of a Victorian house. It has high windows with curtains and blinds and eight comfortable chairs stand on its carpet. Unfortunately, it also contains a large table, two filing cabinets, a projector screen, a flip chart, a portable white board and three boxed resuscitation mannequins. This is also an environment that is not conducive to discussion. Teaching environments are often less than ideal.

It helps to arrive, where possible, before the session to arrange the room and the furniture to the best advantage. The usual arrangements for discussions are to have the chairs arranged in a close circle for an open discussion and in a semi-circle with the leader at the centre, for a closed discussion. Anyone sitting on chairs that have been pulled back tends to be marginalised and should be asked to bring their chairs back into the semi-circle. Sometimes chairs are moved out of alignment, say during coffee break, and this seemingly inconsequential act has implications for the quality of the discussion. If the leader's chair is not symmetrical and his or her field of vision is skewed, some participants at the peripheral blind spots may feel marginalised by a lack of eye contact. Members who do not feel fully part of the group tend to withdraw and cease making contributions. It follows that their learning is also diminished.

STARTING A DISCUSSION

The start of the session will often be the first time that the leader meets the group. It may also be the first time the members have met each other. The first thing to do is to get to know one another. Create enough of a sense of membership to allow a group discussion to function. There are numerous strategies for so doing. For instance, members might be asked to talk, in pairs, for two minutes and take turns reporting on each other to the group at the end. However, this kind of exercise usually gives more information than most people can handle. By the time the third report is reached members often have forgotten the first individual's name and who it was who worked in A & E or was it Urology?

For discussion purposes, names are the most important thing to know and use. Therefore, with a few moments warning, ask each group member to state his or her name and give one other distinctive piece of information. This may be a pet hate or a passion, a favourite railway station or restaurant. Thus we might have Stephen who has a passion for Marmite toast, Carol who hates Opera and so on. A name and a 'handle' are usually enough to begin with. However, at this point it is also useful to ask group members what they want to get out of the discussion, and to record their answers for later reference.

In addition to establishing names and some rapport, introductions also set the session's tone. Whether intentionally or not, the way the introduction is handled tells the group a good deal about the discussion to come. They gain some idea of its mood. Will it be formal or informal? Will it be thoughtful and reflective or lively and sharp?

Above all, will it be helpful and productive. Whatever else is to be conveyed in the introduction, one thing must be made clear and this is that the process will be positive. All contributions will be valued and, whilst it is quite possible to reject ideas, there can be no place for rejecting or devaluing the person. Negative and destructive criticism have no place in a group learning discussion. The third aspect of the introduction is the task and its objectives. The group needs a clear description of the nature of the activity to be undertaken including a statement of the objectives. Once underway, questions of one sort or another form an important teaching strategy.

148

QUESTIONS

Teaching ideas often derive from experiences since pupils and schoolteachers frequently use two types of questions. First there is the 'Who can tell me?' question, when hands shoot up. If the first answer is incorrect then clues are given until someone eventually guessed the word the teacher was looking for. The second kind of question was usually prefaced by a snarled 'You there!'

The questions here have different purposes. Ostensibly, the first, the 'Who can tell me?' question is intended to check the state of the learner's knowledge, although it often ends up as a game in which the learners guess the word in the teacher's head. The second is intended to remind learners that their mental alertness and learning may be checked at any time. The question is used as a means of control. For instance, if the group leader begins by asking questions at one end of the group and progresses systematically to the other, this allows the members to predict when their turn will come and to relax (switch off) when it has passed.

If the group leader poses random questions members have to be alert. A suggested sequence would be to pose the question, then pause for a count of 5 - 7. During this time, do not fix on anyone but scan the group. This gives the group time to think and the questioner time to actively chose someone to question. This works as a way of keeping them alert or giving a 'quiet' member a chance to speak. Then pounce. This pose, pause and pounce formula is extremely useful in groups. Questions can be used in the pursuit of a whole variety of purposes. Interestingly, in teaching, a question is seldom asked because the teacher needs the information requested. Most already know the answer before they ask the question. Thus, when planning a discussion it is important to think about the kinds and purpose of questions to be asked and about what to do with the answers.

Frequently, the question is asked but nothing is done with the answer. Take this case of a group arranged for a closed discussion. The leader completes the introduction and goes on to say: 'Well, as you know, this morning we are going to discuss paediatric basic life support. Have any of you had any first hand experience of this?' Two of the six group members indicate that they have. 'Oh good!' says the leader and goes on to explain what paediatric basic life support involves. There was no attempt to use the answer to find out about and build upon the experience. It is important to be aware of the purpose of asking questions and to have a good idea of how to constructively use the answer. The more the answers are ignored ('Oh good!') the fewer answers will be offered.

PROBLEM-BASED LEARNING

Learning of knowledge, skills, attitudes, or relationships proceeds by stages. Like the medical student memorising anatomical details, we begin by memorising information. The next stage in acquiring medical knowledge involves interpretation. This requires the student to place anatomic details within a physiological context and explain them as part of a functioning system. The third stage is analysis. This requires the ability to mentally manipulate physiological systems, to test hypotheses, and produce a diagnosis. Synthesis involves using all that prior knowledge to produce a patient management plan, which ultimately can be evaluated. Evaluation is the final stage in knowledge acquisition.

149

Problem-based learning is a means of running these stages concurrently and has been a feature in education for more than thirty years. In postgraduate and continuing medical education, it could be argued that any practitioner who identifies problems with his patients and sets about finding solutions through analytical reading or discussions with colleagues is participating in problem-based learning and to that extent it is hardly a new concept. However, its importance and relevance in undergraduate education has only been recognised in the last ten years. Students are now encouraged to develop problem-solving techniques from the outset, to promote the development of intrinsic motivation and reflection.

Typically, this small group model, guided by a tutor, is used to facilitate the investigation of clinical problems. Three major principles are involved in the process:

- The activation of prior knowledge requiring a certain level of background expertise.
- Learners must feel that the case is real and is in a relevant context.
- Identification of a problem or problems with pursuit of a line of enquiry, reflection and elaboration on the information obtained. This implies discussion with colleagues, tutors, other specialists, and/or reading around the subject.

This technique has a number of drawbacks. It has been criticised because the outcomes can be too open-ended and inexperienced students may not be able to distil the problem sufficiently to achieve worthwhile objectives in a finite amount of time. Some of their analytical skills can be developed by using written case studies. However, as one of the main aims of problem-based learning is working with real patients, these should be used sparingly and only in the initial stages. More senior trainees, such as postgraduate medical staff on a ward, benefit most from the problem-based model, since this approach should underpin everyday work activity. The relevance of this to teaching on business rounds is discussed in more detail in Chapter Eleven.

Teachers in problem-based learning for undergraduates must be more than simple facilitators. Where necessary, they must be tutors, guiding the direction of learning. Fulfilment of this role comes about by the asking of pertinent thought-provoking questions and guiding discussions integrating various learning issues and finally, by determining the path for future exploration.

Most formal studies have been at an undergraduate level and suggest that problem-based learning is both enjoyable and encourages self-directed learning. Perhaps, not surprisingly, it appears to work best for cognitive learning and is not as useful for practical skills. Also, although it would seem to produce a more enquiring mind, there is no proof of better outcomes as far as the present undergraduate or, indeed, postgraduate examination systems are concerned. Therefore, problem-based learning should be seen as another useful technique for motivating learners at all levels, but is certainly not a panacea for the whole of training curriculum.

For continuing medical education, it is the *sine qua non* of the reflective practitioner. As such, its use should be encouraged at all levels of undergraduate and postgraduate training. It should become a routine part of medical practice.

Clearly, if learners need to progress through a number of stages, the group leader needs to know where the group members are. This indicates the leader's role and the purpose of a group process. Further, there is little point in generating discussion at the level of analysis or synthesis if the learner is still at the memorising or interpreting stage. Therefore, the teacher needs to be skilled in organising teaching episodes, not least of which is the response to statements and questions from the group.

Two things follow from learners' progress through these stages. First, the leader's awareness of the approximate stage group members have reached may give the first real purpose for the questioning. Secondly, if the learner is still at the memorising or interpreting stage, there is little point in asking questions at the level of analysis or synthesis. Types of question at the five levels are given below.

Given that we now have some idea of the appropriate cognitive level for questions, it still must be decided, for instance, whether they should be directed, whether open or closed, simple or complex. That is, should the question be put to a specific individual to answer, or to the whole group? Unless group members know their individual capabilities, and unless all individuals are to be asked at some stage, then it is better to question the group as a whole. Should an individual be unable or reluctant to answer, negativity enters into the proceedings. This can be intensified if the leader asks vague or complex questions. Assuming the cognitive level is right and undirected, simple, open questions have been asked the next task is to respond to the answers.

LISTENING AND RESPONDING

Whether in open, closed or workshop discussion it is difficult to overemphasise the importance of listening. Often, there will be only a few short phrases, sometimes only a word or two upon which to base decisions about the most appropriate response for that individual and for the group. The leader must listen, interpret and make decisions about where to go next. It is important to be an active listener, displaying through posture, gesture and expression that one is listening. An appropriate question has been asked and a good answer obtained, what next? There are numerous ways to respond at this point. Answers from group members might be:

- Reflected back to the individual – 'What do you think?'
- Reflected to the group – 'What do the rest of you think?'
- Questioned – 'Would that necessarily follow?' ' Why do you say that?'
- Developed – 'So? What would that imply?'
- Directed to another member – 'Isn't that what you were saying earlier, Ian?'
- Answered – with fact or opinion or 'I don't know, I'm not sure about that'. This usually obliges the speaker to continue.

Most of these responses would be used in open discussion. In a closed discussion questions from members to the leader are more likely to be given straight answers or to be turned to the leader's agenda. Below are two examples of discussion, one closed, and one open. This should indicate the importance of leader responses.

The first example is a description of an academic course for general practitioners. The group were to have a closed discussion on research methods using ear infections as a focus. There were four GPs plus Steve, a faculty member who was to act as a leader.

Steve	OK, what do we know about ear infections?
Tony	Had an interesting chap in the other day with glue-ear.
Steve	Anyone keep any records or compile any statistics on this kind of thing?
Simon	We get lots. I had two little chaps in this week, one whose problem had cleared up. I had a look in his ears and the grommets were still there...
Steve	Grommets, what do we know about the history of grommets? It's very interesting if you look at the statistics you can see an enormous rise in the use of grommets and yet there has been no evaluation of them whatsoever. How is it that we can use something without knowing whether it works?
Julie	But they do work in some cases, that's the point, it must be worth a try. I use them whenever...
Steve	Julie, I want to bring you in with your own experiences at the rele vant points, but first I think we should have a look at the Friedman and Sacks paper...

The group go on to discuss the paper but do not return to personal experiences. Eventually Steve concludes in a rather pleased way with:

Steve	Good. You've actually done precisely what I hoped you would, that is, you've concluded that the evidence for grommets is mixed, we have no real evidence that the grommets have any effect.

There are some problems here. Steve ignores Tony's contribution, picks out what he wants from Simon and puts Julie on hold. It is a successful closed discussion in that it is tightly controlled and reaches the point Steve was aiming for. As a group members' learning experience it was probably much less so. Steve might have begun by asking and perhaps recording each member's experiences. Then he might attempt to discern commonalties or patterns within those experiences. From these, the group might have explored how these patterns could be identified and measured. This would lead into a consideration of what research involves and the methods of achieving it.

The second example is taken from a course on consultation skills for the GP Part of the course is designed to allow the members to reflect upon their attitudes to patients. In this group there are six group members plus Sarah, one of the course organisers, who acts as leader. The topic for this open discussion is 'difficult patients'.

Sarah	What kind of patients makes you cross?
James	Aggressive patients tend to make me angry.

Lynn	*Why?*
James	*It's a natural thing, to react, isn't it?*
Lynn	*Do you take it personally?*
James	*Yes, of course I do…*
Javid	*What about manipulative patients, people wanting sick notes when there's nothing wrong with them? Don't you feel you are being used?*
Helen	*No, I think it's more than that, it's the only way some patients can get what they want.*
Javid	*But by getting what they want they are taking control and that's what makes me angry.*
Sarah	*Why is it so important to be in control?*
Javid	*Because otherwise they don't want my advice, they just want a pre-scription, they tell me what they want and I become just a pen pusher for the patients.*
Bryan	*The patients who make me angry are those who don't co-operate in the process of making them well and that's really another aspect of control.*
Sarah	*Let's take this issue of control a little further. How do we normally control the consultation? Paula?*

Sarah is prepared to let the discussion flow as it is identifying a topic, which eventually becomes 'control'. Once she recognises it as a good topic she focuses the discussion 'Why is it important to be in control?' And again, 'How do we normally control the consultation? At that point, aware that Paula is the only member not to have contributed so far, she invites her to speak. This discussion appears to be more productive than the previous example. However, we should be clear about this - the comparison is between two group leaders, Steve and Sarah and not between discussion styles. Discussion can be ruined by negative responses, such as:

- 'That is absolute rubbish.'
- 'You're actually touching on a very important area here, but you're just groping around.'
- 'I'd have thought that was obvious.'
- 'I've already given you the answer to this one but you didn't recognise it.'
- 'I thought I'd already dealt with this question in my recent paper in….'

SUMMARY AND TERMINATION

Throughout the discussion it may be necessary to take stock. The group leader must take responsibility for this by reviewing the arguments to date and identifying, common threads and themes. This may happen several times during the discussion. It certainly will do so at the end. Enough time must be left for this activity. Before the discussion is summarised it is usual to ask for any further comments or questions. Discussions that tail-off feel unsatisfactory, perhaps because, as in many educational encounters, it is what is taken away that matters. Summaries provide structure and feedback - both essential elements in learning. Structure comes from the identification and classification of common elements (the arguments for or against), it reduces detail and helps to make connections. Feedback gives the individual information about how his or her performance was perceived by others. It is also essential for learning.

Having summarised, the leader will probably give details of the next session and thank everyone for their contribution. Terminating a session is simple enough but can go wrong. Generally, doctors are expert at terminating consultations and know that it is up to them to give the patient a clear and definite signal that the consultation is over. Discussions require the same kind of signal - stand up, turn away, pack your papers etc.

PROBLEMS

There are always problems in running discussion groups. Some are more likely to occur than others, these are listed below.

—*A question is asked but no one can give an answer.*

This suggests that either they do not understand the question or a blank spot has been hit in their recollection. In either case, it may be necessary to rephrase the question in a more closed form. As a last resort, a yes/no question can be used and the discussion gradually opened up from there.

—*One member of the group starts to rush in with an answer every time.*

Stop this person by suggesting that it would be good to hear a range of opinions, then go on to someone else, before going back to them for a second opinion. Deliberately, avoid eye contact or hold up a hand as soon as they start to speak and invite a contribution from elsewhere. Use names to request answers or indicate who has the floor.

—*The answer is too long and elaborate.*

Interrupt, thank the speaker for their answer, but explain that, for discussion purposes an answer in a more usable form is needed then ask if someone can supply it in a succinct way.

—*The answer appears to have absolutely nothing to do with the topic being discussed.*

This can be a 'show stopper' as no one can perceive the relevance of the ideas offered. The answer could be translated into something useful ('This is obviously a reference to…') But probably it is best to go back to the group member and seek clarification.

—*The issue under discussion is the process of learning but the group continually returns to clinical matters.*

After some initial steering it is best to stop the group and remind them of the brief. Restart the discussion in a positive way.

—*A group member offers critical and rather destructive comments on another's contribution.*

It is important to intervene and ask the individual for suggestions for improvement and to remind the group that positive comments are most productive.

—*One member of the group offers no answers and seems not to be participating.*

It is possible for a non-contributing group member to be gaining much from the discussion. On the other hand, this particular individual may want to contribute but be reluctant for a variety of reasons. He or she can be given the opportunity to contribute through direct, simple questions which also check the individual's experiences in relation to the topic under discussion.

—One or more members of the group provide negative and possibly aggressive responses to questions. ('I really can't see the point of this…Do you expect us to take this seriously?')

This is the destroyer at work. It is someone who already knows about teaching and learning and views the serious study of education as an extravagant waste of time.

With such individuals, remember that the content of their comment is entirely unimportant, it is simply a vehicle for being negative. If you provide a satisfactory answer to their first question their next will be just as negative. Hence, the aggression has to be tackled - 'That was a very negative statement, do you have a problem with this activity?' At which point the hostile member may well claim that 'Discussion is a waste of time.' The group can be enlisted to discuss the value of discussion as a learning medium. If the reluctant individual is not drawn into the discussion but persists in making destructive comments, terminate the discussion, remove the individual for a 'quiet word' and reconvene without that person. The group cannot function as a learning mechanism whilst it contains individuals who are bent on disrupting it.

By no means, does this exhaust the possible problems encountered in discussion groups, but it gives some idea of what to expect and some suggestions for coping. Other ways of going wrong may be revealed by an evaluation.

EVALUATION

Usually, it is courses that are evaluated not individual components such as discussion groups. Nevertheless, there may be some benefit in attempting to assess the value of the session.

It should be possible to devise and use quick fill-in check sheets asking about levels of satisfaction and so on. However, these may be cumbersome and the kind of information yielded may not be particularly useful. Evaluation can be done verbally. One way would be to return to the question asked at the beginning, namely, 'What do you hope to get out of this session?' Remind the group of the answers they gave (they may be on a flip chart or white board) and ask each whether they have achieved what they hoped for from the discussion. Alternatively, ask each to say one thing of value which they had learned and one way in which this discussion could have been improved. This verbal approach provides useful information and seems an appropriate way of evaluating the process of discussion.

CONCLUSION

Small group teaching is not a panacea or a corrective for the supposed ills of the lecture. Like the lecture, the value of small group work depends upon the appropriateness of the topic and on the group leader's knowledge, skill and enthusiasm. With a good topic and a skilled leader, small groups can provide all the stimulus of colleague discussion directed towards specific and worthwhile objectives.

CHAPTER 11
Teaching with Patients

BRIAN JOLLY, DUNCAN HARRIS
& RODNEY PEYTON

INTRODUCTION

THIS CHAPTER is about undergraduate and postgraduate teaching in the clinical environment. We will approach this task from the perspectives developed in the first section and, in particular, those cultivated by the chapters on learning by adults.

Teaching in the clinical environment is often called 'Bedside Teaching'. This term is now too restrictive for several reasons. The trend towards shorter hospital stays and the marked increase in day procedures means patients are rarely 'in bed' in hospital long enough for this phrase to encapsulate all those things that concern us. In addition, a number of other important learning environments are excluded by the term. These include outpatients, outreach clinics, and general practice which increasingly is the prime setting for holistic care coupled with long term continuity in patient management. In this chapter, therefore, we will focus on the teacher's collaboration with the patient and the learner or trainee to create a useful learning environment.

Learning in the clinical environment is essential to becoming a fully qualified doctor. It offers a unique blend of university and work place for postgraduate training. The clinical environment, a diverse, pulsating and frequently hectic one, offers the potential for attaining skills in clinical history-taking, patient examination and diagnosis and management of various conditions that include problem solving and decision making. It is the one place *par excellance* where relationships can develop between the patient and the medical team, whether on an individual or group basis. Hence, it fosters the development of communication skills with both patients and colleagues.

It is vital that this environment is used appropriately to enable the doctor in training to learn those things that clinical surroundings can best foster. It also must be used dynamically in the sense of establishing a good learning milieu promoting interaction between learner, teacher and patient. Also, the trainers can observe students and trainees in a practical as opposed to a theoretical setting and senior staff can demonstrate their professionalism, not just in terms of knowledge and skills, but also in their attitude towards caring for patients.

Therefore, it is important for teachers to 'walk their talk' so that what they say and what they do coincide in the working environment. For instance, teachers should pay more than lip-service to good practice in such things as maintaining sterility, barrier nursing and the maintenance of a quiet rest hour for patients. Even beyond these clinical concepts, the demonstration by senior staff of self-discipline, punctuality, a caring attitude and flexibility in working practice to accommodate patients, other colleagues and staff, can have a profound effect on the future conduct of those who are beginning to make their way up the professional ladder.

Many problems in teaching with patients come from mismatches between the environment and expectations about what objectives can actually be achieved. For example, many clinical teachers on the ward, drift towards activities more appropriate to the lecture theatre or seminar room and designed to impart detailed factual knowledge. So the clinical context is used for things it cannot achieve. Often, aspects of the context are mismanaged or ignored. Learners can be turned off unless totally involved in some activity and provided with instant feedback since human attention span is short. We also know that the learner's capacity to process new information is affected by tiredness, engendered by over-long rounds, or previous nights on-call. Yet, commonly on a two to three hour ward round the most active participant is the senior consultant or registrar. The potential for the others to be distracted is vast, especially if standing for prolonged periods of time, particularly in an open ward. Standing also emphasises difference in height which may be intimidating for smaller trainees and introduce problems into group dynamics. Maximum involvement of trainees and, where appropriate, of the patient has to be cultivated to maintain everyone's interest in and commitment to a learning session.

Cases do not occur in a sensible or logical order and there is an obvious necessity for being opportunistic in clinical teaching. However, some element of planning is required.

It is therefore useful to review what we require in terms of adult learning. We need to:

- Recognise that the role of a patient in the learning process is determined by having clear goals for the session.
- Recognise the capacity of the learner in terms of existing knowledge, skills and attitudes.
- Maintain personal motivation.
- Make learning meaningful.
- Actively involve learners.
- Focus on experience and allow learners to reflect on that experience.
- Give feedback on trainees' skills and development.

In the remainder of this chapter, we will look at each of these features in terms of the clinical environment and suggest steps to use the strengths and avoid the weaknesses inherent in this activity. Unfortunately, many of the things assumed to be happening in clinical teaching either do not occur at all or do so with less frequency than we would like. However, note that the most fully researched environment is the hospital ward with an overwhelming concentration on the activities of the clinical teacher. Thus, some of the disadvantages found with clinical teaching in hospitals will not occur in other contexts.

The two most common ward teaching scenarios are the teaching round and the business round. Both are variants of the small group teaching process reviewed more extensively in Chapter Ten. The particular characteristics of the types of ward round will now be discussed.

TEACHING ROUNDS

An historical perspective can be useful in guiding us toward better practice. Believe it or not, clinical teaching is a relatively recent phenomenon. For the four centuries preceding the 17th, most of a physician's preparation for practice was by reading, not by clinical contact with patients. However, as science and empiricism developed, simple reliance on printed knowledge was threatened by the need to verify theoretical assertions in terms of patient outcome. This created both clinical work and clinical education.

Originating in Italy, and nurtured by early Austrian and Dutch clinical schools, the style of medical and patient-based teaching was moulded by those clinical or theoretical orientations dominating the academic community at the time. Both traditions were, and still are, engaged in a perennial tension. Should the primary focus for medical education be the patient's needs or should it be demands for scientific rigour? In practice, this debate influenced where learning activity took place, the clinic, or the library/laboratory? John Abernethy, an early founder of British clinical education, said:

'The hospital is the only proper College in which to rear a true disciple of Aesculapius.'

However, in 1858, the divorce between academic and practical aspects of medicine was enshrined by the General Medical Council in the U.K. as the whole country's statutory educational model. This rift between theory and practice was granted a decree absolute in 1910 in North America. There, Abraham Flexner reviewed and effectively charted a new course for medical education for the next century. Briefly, his review resulted in a comprehensive increase in the emphasis on scientific, single discipline-oriented, predominantly laboratory-based studies in the undergraduate medical curriculum.

THE NATURE OF A TEACHING ROUND

Teaching rounds are inclined to be formal episodes with a specific time set aside for the study of an isolated case or number of cases. The time is usually committed on a regular basis, and thus, there is ample opportunity to plan in advance. They can be organised to follow a teaching syllabus. They fit best with undergraduate or early postgraduate education, since these tend to be exam orientated. In general terms, it is the disease process that becomes the central theme, with history-taking and clinical examination the starting point from which discussion can develop. The teaching tends to be theoretically based with a lesser emphasises on practicality.

THE PATIENT'S ROLE

In this context, it is easy to see how the patient might be forgotten. Therefore, thought should be given to the way the patient's presence enhances the learning episode. Some clinical teaching manuals hardly mention the patient's role. Various studies of patients' views about involvement in teaching provide some useful guidelines:

- On a teaching round, the objective is educational and often of little direct benefit to the patient. The patient's permission should be sought in advance if he or she is going to be presented for teaching rather than clinical management purposes, either to you by the trainees or vice versa.
- Patients should be told the main aim of their involvement and the aspects of the history or finding most pertinent to your goals.
- Unless patients are anxious, or in physical discomfort, they may actually prefer to remain for the discussion, as long as it does not touch on detailed personal and social data.
- Consideration should be given to the surrounding environment, including the ward layout, in order to afford the patient maximum privacy. Sensitive issues should be discussed out of the rest of the ward's hearing. It may be more suitable for the patient to be examined in a side room.
- Communicating with the patient about his or her condition should feature in the discussion. Also, the patient is the best person to detail the effects of the disease, and its interaction with his or her lifestyle.
- Afterwards, senior staff may need to debrief the patient about the teaching session. Thus, any necessary explanations can be given, worries addressed and misconceptions immediately corrected.

Such preparation will provide a more relaxed atmosphere in which to teach and get patients on your side.

STARTING WITH CLEAR GOALS

One important historical feature of clinical medicine influenced the evolution of clinical education. This was the notion of the doctor's personal responsibility for the patient. This gave rise to the apprenticeship systems dominating European clinical education for several hundred years. While having very useful influences on patient care, provision of role models, supervision and ethical practice, it has tended to obscure the need to have clear goals for learners. After all, an *apprentice* learning a craft has been around for years. Bits and pieces could be slotted into place rather like a patchwork quilt. However, this is no longer so easy, although many teachers carry on as if it were.

The most recent directives on defining goals have come from the Association of American Medical Colleges report on 'Physicians for the 21st Century', and in the UK, from the GMC and Calman reports. These identified general principles about the role, value, and appropriate structure for clinical education that included:

- Faculties or Colleges should collectively specify the clinical knowledge, skills, values, and attitudes that learners need.
- They should describe in more detail the clinical settings appropriate for this clinical education.
- Teachers should have adequate preparation and time to guide and supervise trainees.
- Clinical performance should be regularly assessed.

Part of the process of starting with clear goals is thinking about what clinical teaching can and cannot do. That is, to choose goals and objectives appropriate to the advantages of the setting and to what learners might, or might not, have experienced prior to arriving with your unit or practice. Even when asked to teach at short notice, a few minutes taken to think out a clear structure before the teaching begins reaps large rewards in the efficiency of the teaching process.

Most clinicians would agree that one of clinical education's main goals, whether hospital or practice-based, is to allow the trainee to become competent in identifying, recording and analysing symptoms presented in individual cases as a basis for diagnosis and treatment.

The fulfilment of this task is the goal of teaching with patients. Thus, when using patients, it is important to do a number of things to clarify what is being taught and why:

- For each session, choose a topic appropriate to the trainees' needs and to time available. Negotiate objectives with the trainees (perhaps in an earlier meeting) and agree on what they should be able to do or know after the session, that they could not do before. Try to point out to trainees the session's relevance, goals and objectives within the context of their overall experience. Stress the main points. Take no more than 5 minutes to do this.
- Plan to maximise teaching time with the patient. Do as much preparation as possible away from the patient so that essential clinical tasks can be accomplished with them. Do not waste clinical time by giving lectures, tutorials, or question and answer sessions that could be given elsewhere or at another time.
- Before the session, consider the trainees' knowledge level and whether it can be enhanced by pre-reading or perhaps a micro-teaching session for five to ten

minutes in the clinical room prior to the bedside meeting. The trainer or one of the trainees and can run this. It offers an excellent opportunity to allow more senior trainees or brighter students to utilise their knowledge and enhance their presentation skills. At the same time, they can help to raise the knowledge threshold of the rest of the group.

- If appropriate, ensure that learners have a hand-out or a reference on general principles for material they need but that the session cannot cover. Refer to it frequently, and in subsequent sessions ask trainees to recall or demonstrate ideas from it.

160

By doing these things you significantly improve the framework of your clinical teaching compared to the norm especially at undergraduate level. For example, studies monitoring educational activity in hospital settings found evidence that time devoted to clinical activity was erratic or even non-existent. It ranged from 0% to 25% of students' time on the ward. Hence, it would be even better if the session could actually meet the trainees' needs.

Even in the new order, teaching rounds continue to be a focus for education, but their organisation needs to provide adequate support for bedside teaching and development of clinical skills. In the USA, Mattern found that of six attending physician teams studied, only three visited the bedside for educational purposes. Other studies of ward rounds *in action* found that discussion often focused on minutiae, or on esoteric or scientific aspects of the case not amenable to bedside investigation. In one study, topics most appropriate to ward-round teaching (patient examination and doctor-patient communication), occupied less than 10% of the round. Others have shown that within teaching rounds two-thirds of the time was spent in the conference room, one-quarter in hallways and only approximately 10% at the bedside. This is compounded by the fact that the availability of clinical experience has decreased in the last 10 years, especially in inner city hospitals.

In summary, the clinical teaching environment is the best place to concentrate on the clinical skills of doctor/patient interaction, physical examination and history-taking. Long erudite conferences around the patient or afterwards on complications, similar cases, and underlying mechanisms may be appropriate at some stage. However, they may waste or ignore the most precious resource available - the physical presence of the patient.

RECOGNISE AND EMPLOY
EXISTING KNOWLEDGE AND SKILLS

Reviews have attempted to identify a number of features that seem to contribute to trainee satisfaction and good clinical learning. These include a responsibility for, and contribution towards, some aspects of their learning and teaching pitched at the right level for the learner's degree of experience. However, 'teaching' ward rounds often have little opportunity for students to contribute. They are more likely to be on the receiving end of low level knowledge questions from the trainer.

Indeed, some studies have found undergraduate and postgraduate student contribution to teaching and business rounds to be even less than that in lectures with student input being significant only in patient management conferences and morning reports. Moreover, the teaching content is frequently unconnected with patient care, clinical skills, doctor/patient communication or management. Some ways to involve the learners are listed below.

Another problem to be overcome is that learners have rarely undertaken common learning experiences. The clinical environment is not like a university classroom where most of the class receive at least the same set of stimuli, lectures, handouts, laboratory experiments and so on. In medicine, even if individual trainees or students have encountered the same clinical conditions, they are likely to have done so in patients who have dissimilar personalities, symptoms, anatomies, racial features, and social backgrounds. Certainly, they will have experienced these diseases in different orders and in varying degrees. All of these factors will have a profound effect on how the content of medicine is perceived and on how learners manoeuvre their way through it. Therefore:

1. Try to find out what the learners already know about the patient or topic. This will help you pitch the session appropriately. Since they are likely to be reticent about sharing ignorance, set ground rules which allow them to do this. Do not ridicule lack of knowledge, but encourage good guesses and rough outlines, reinforcing their accurate understanding and filling in gaps.

2. Try to get them to identify their own needs or worries in the area - it will help you choose appropriate objectives. One way to do this is to get a small group to go away to identify what they do or do not know about and come back 20 minutes later with a summary. This takes you (the experienced know-it-all) out of the way and allows them to sort out a better approach than would have emerged on a packed round. It also allows admission of what might be embarrassing individual needs, to be subsumed into an aggregated need. During the 20 minutes you can be busy with some other work.

   Another way to set about it is by getting them to summarise their collective experience of other patients of the type you are going to see, in terms of symptoms, diagnosis, and management.

   A further alternative allows individuals to quickly recognise their own weaknesses with respect to a case. Get each team member to jot down their first thoughts about a patient and then discuss them with another member before doing a 'question round'. This allows individuals to mask any deficiencies they have from public (your) view, while promoting good teamwork and individual reflection on their true needs.

   All of these activities can be done away from the patient. It may be neither useful nor desirable for them to be involved for the whole period. Accordingly, it may be more appropriate to begin the round in a clinical room, discussing theory in a practical context. Following this, the group can meet at the bedside in order to practice clinical skills from history-taking to examination. Depending on circumstances, the group may withdraw to discuss test results, consider the various differential diagnoses, problem-solve, and review possible management methods.

3. Using and maintaining group size. Another important method of making clinical teaching more active is in using and maintaining group size. Most medical teachers remember with affection the clinical teachers that taught them well when they were junior. What they may have forgotten is the number of times they could not see, could not hear, were distracted, were called away, had no one to teach them - or perhaps they will remember it only too vividly. The clinical environment is not learner- or teacher-friendly. It needs to be made so.

Do not try to teach a group that is bigger than three to four learners per patient. 'Impossible!', you say. 'Today's health care system is too...' you add. But this work load does not mean that you have to teach the entire team at the same patient. One of the most effective outpatients' sessions was run by a consultant who sat on a chair in the middle of the clinic, while all of his team from registrar to student dealt individually with patients, consulting with him only when needed. Each team member had about 10-15 minutes of one on one teaching in the session. The patients were all seen. The students took longest and needed the most help, but were given the easiest patients (follow-ups and routine consultations), but all patients saw a qualified doctor at some stage. Of course, with the UK Patients' Charter such a system may be unacceptable. Yet the principle of breaking up the group into smaller units and checking on their progress is a good one. Below we have a few tricks for doing this:

- Using pairs and other group sizes. Rather than have everybody look at the same patient, send pairs off to examine and consult with different individual patients and then report back with their findings. Use this time to follow up on weaker learners - maybe checking on their examination technique or other clinical skills.
- The more junior the learners, the less content they will assimilate in one session. They will not be able to concentrate on everything in one round or outpatient session. Break juniors' tasks up into manageable units. Do not require everything from everyone - there will not be time for this anyway. For example ask different people to demonstrate different bits of the examination technique, rather than the whole process. Do not tell them beforehand which part of the technique they will have to do until just before you need it. You can structure early history-taking sessions by asking one student to take the past medical history and, when he or she has finished, inviting another to take the family history and a third to review systems etc. Other learners or trainees can be encouraged to give constructive feedback.
- Demonstrate clinical skills to a maximum of four people at a time. Get seniors to teach juniors rather than trying to teach everything yourself. The teaching of clinical skills, such as catheter insertion, is more appropriately undertaken elsewhere than on the ward, for instance in a skills laboratory. Some techniques such as taking blood pressure and using ophthalmoscopes can be practised by trainees on each other. Only when a basic level of skill has been achieved should they practice on patients.

In a wider context, for example, after the Calman reforms of postgraduate educa-

162

tion in the UK, and certainly after the GMC recommendations for undergraduates, it may no longer make organisational sense to deliver learning by attachment to a single 'firm'. Also, research has consistently suggested that work-related, patient-based experience is more frequent and prolonged in district, community or other non-teaching/non university-affiliated hospitals, although most researchers do not directly suggest why this should be the case.

A number of factors could contribute. There may be fewer students per patient, more staff time per student, or perhaps more patients with a range of conditions being present on one ward, as opposed to having a number of patients with similar conditions relating to the activities of a specialised unit. Similarly, more appropriate teaching units may be ward (as opposed to firm) based, 'Day Surgery' and Outpatients or General Practice/Health Centres where each learner sees whoever is available or whichever team is using the facilities during their attachments. This is challenging for younger students, especially undergraduates, who may have to cross systems boundaries with every new patient. The pace of early learning will need to be slowed down and the patients used more as a focus for individual learner activity rather than as the basic 'fodder' of a disciplinary approach.

For postgraduate trainees it should not be a problem, but negotiation of goals and objectives suitable to the environments on offer must be done first. Certainly, new and more appropriate organisational frameworks for teaching will need to be developed, but it is not yet clear what these might be. Whatever develops, attachments will need clear and agreed goals, as well as trainees who take most of the responsibility for their own learning, and planned and appropriate use of the richness of the clinical environment.

MAINTAIN PERSONAL MOTIVATION AND MAKE LEARNING MEANINGFUL

To a certain extent, negotiating objectives, telling learners what these are and pointing out their relevance within the clinical context will help make learning more meaningful. Other specific ways of approaching this issue include:

1. Using time appropriately. One way to do this is by varying the stimulus. A mix of skills, knowledge-based and interpersonal activities for 30 minutes each will be better than an hour (or more) long session of only one activity.

2. Use a location appropriate to the task. Do not talk in a corridor or a teaching room if the topic needs a patient for demonstration purposes. A long question and answer session on Diverticulitis may best be done away from the bedside. These ideas may seem obvious but research shows that such self-evident issues are frequently ignored.

3. You will have to use educational activities that are most engaging for the learners or trainees in areas where there are most distractions (ends of wards, hallways, corridors and labs). Do not attempt monologues and content input in these settings. Use one or more of the following:

   —*Individual tasks* in which, for example, learners have to work out a management strategy for a patient or a diagnostic approach.

—*Brainstorming*, which can be used in difficult cases or where the appropriate management is unclear. Everybody is asked to contribute ideas with no penalty for apparently inappropriate or idiosyncratic ones. (They may turn out to be creatively useful.)

—*Jotting down thoughts* is useful when reflection/thinking time is needed and you want everyone to contribute. Everyone has to think and write down one or two conclusions about an issue. For example, what issues about post-operative care are we confronted with by Mr. Jones' newly diagnosed Altzheimers disease?

—*Paired or snowballing discussion* is an extension of the above. Each person discusses their initial thoughts with another, and then maybe with another pair (i.e., in a foursome), and so on. Conclusions and ideas are refined at each stage.

4. Feedback is an essential component of maintaining motivation – see below.

5. Either postpone the session or set the learners a task they can accomplish in the time if you cannot turn up or are delayed. Make sure these tasks are followed up when you do eventually surface. If you are interrupted and called away, set the learners a task to be done while you are gone; make it easy, doable and checkable on your return.

6. When demonstrating skills use the four-step approach outlined in Chapter Twelve, which we will briefly mention here:

—After briefly orientating the student, both about the skill and what will happen in the session, perform a real-time demonstration of the skill with no commentary.

—Then perform again with an explanation getting the learners to observe.

—Ask one or more learners to talk you through the skill while you demonstrate.

—Ask one or more learners to describe and demonstrate the skill to you.

7. Provide a good role model for learners. This is important because students and doctors in training often see examples of bad-practice that they know not to copy. They need to supplement these with roles and competencies at which they can aim. Involving patients in the teaching process, by asking them sensible questions at appropriate points and even allowing them to contribute to the teaching is a useful adjunct to clinical activity. After all, they will know many things about their disease that junior students may not. Most bed-based, patients will need to be briefed, but it is a very useful technique in the outpatient setting.

8. Provide a supportive atmosphere to learning. Do not humiliate juniors, especially in front of patients. If someone makes a bad error, point it out briefly and see him or her after the session. Try to get them to identify what the problem was first before gently suggesting that they might need further activities to remedy it. Use the four-step feedback model described on page 28.

9. It may also be necessary to control the behaviour of your team's senior members and encourage them not to stifle those their junior. It is important to impart knowledge not merely declare it.

164

ACTIVELY INVOLVE LEARNERS

Having attended nearly 150 clinical sessions during several clinical teaching research projects, we believe watching paint dry to be more entertaining than a ward round or outpatient session wherein learners or trainees get to do nothing. Then there is the operating session in which the main focus of their attention is to hold open the chest wall. From the student's perspective there is very little point in much of this so-called 'activity'. Yet activity is essential for learning. Here we suggest some ways of maximising it.

1. Ask questions frequently, wait for the answers, and do not answer them yourself! This is a simple seldom obeyed rule. It has been shown that 'good' teachers ask questions rather than give students answers. In a busy session, because people need thinking time, you may have to wait for what seems like an interminable length of time (up to 10 seconds) for some answers. They may have to work the answer out, while you 'know' it! Unanswered questions may need to be passed on to another learner. Totally blank faces, even after a long wait or bouncing it to others, mean you may need to ask a simpler question, but don't answer it or the original question yourself.

2. Make sure your questions are relevant and important. Don't ask trivial questions and then wonder why the students don't appear to know anything.

3. Ask open questions first. For example: 'Tell me about the important anatomy of the neck in relation to this thyroidectomy' will be of more use than 'where is the recurrent laryngeal nerve?' This is because the first question allows more answers and will not be so easily or exhaustively answered by one student. You have more information to work with.

4. When learners or trainees respond, try to get them or others to evaluate the answers before passing judgement yourself. Give praise for good answers, and allow the individual and/or group to critique bad ones. Use supportive language such as, 'Any other suggestions to improve the answer?' One extremely important question is 'So what?' The thrust of the question is to encourage the learners to think about their responses in a clinically active way.

5. Get learners to do things as frequently as possible rather than just stand around and listen. If the pulses have not been done, ask a learner to do them and watch closely. If something needs writing down on paper or the board get a student to do it. If there are verbose or dominant learners in the group getting them to be scribe for a while is an aid to keeping them quiet. Unfortunately, scribing can be quite boring, so it's not recommended as a learning tool. To be useful such tasks need to fit with some learning plan. Examining patients, taking histories and so on are probably more useful.

6. Give mini-projects requiring further study at the end of a session. For example, these could include, reading specific papers, arranging report-back sessions, requiring patient summaries or discharge notes, auditing and so on. If you make these homework tasks relevant to the cases you have seen, but do not tell learners or trainees during the session what the projects will be or to whom

they will be given, you will be surprised at their attentiveness during sessions. Make sure you follow these projects up when completed or attention will wane.

7. Every few weeks, reserve one part of a session to discuss difficult cases or topics troubling learners. Take an evidence-based slant on issues and encourage learners to review the literature on these topics.

FEEDBACK

Most early research on clinical settings concentrated almost entirely on the characteristics of the teacher. Later work has highlighted the need to look at the whole clinical environment and at student input. Six major factors in student satisfaction with clinical teaching have been identified:

1. feedback to students
2. clinical exposure
3. staff-student relationships
4. organisation and delivery of teaching
5. involvement with the business of the firm
6. the degree of acuteness of the medicine experienced.

The most important of these factors was feedback to students. The need for feedback in learning has been supported by numerous studies. The value perceived in showing personal interest in learners or trainees, reviewing histories and supervising physical examinations is also highlighted. Senior teachers consistently overestimate how frequently they undertake certain teaching activities, especially those they value highly. Many senior staff members do not regularly give appropriate feedback.

In this respect, it is also useful to make a few points about widespread learning and teaching methods and feedback:

1. Giving feedback on history taking and patient examination requires direct observation. This is because case presentation is a very common method of teaching used frequently on ward rounds. It may be very good for checking that learners or trainees have sought all the required information but it provides no feedback on the way learners take the history or carry out the examination. The latter requires direct scrutiny of those skills. At undergraduate level, such observation may be frequent while for postgraduates, occasional usage may be sufficient. The important issue is that to give feedback on a skill or capacity requires preliminary observation of that skill or capacity. Trainees should be assessed on what they can do, not just on what they say they can do or have done.

2. Either way, feedback is essential. This should be organised along the lines espoused in Chapter Two:

   • Ask for self-perceptions about their state, rather than their skills (how did the learner feel, were they nervous, etc.).
   • Ask the trainee for examples of things they thought they did well.
   • Follow with things you or others (if involved) thought they did well.
   • Then ask the learner to describe possible improvements (being very specific with alternative suggestions).

- Next, contribute those from yourself or others.
- Finally, provide a mini summary of points for improvement. No more than three would be recommended. You may give the summary or ask a member of the group or the individual trainee.

FOCUS ON EXPERIENCE AND SUMMARISE

1. At the end of each teaching session review what has gone on and check that the objectives have been met. Learners can assist in this by reporting to you what you have covered. Ask patients for their perceptions.
2. Make a note of those objectives that have been covered and any that have not.
3. Ask for any remaining questions.
4. Try to summarise by reviewing what has been done and achieved in the session. For example, 'Today we have spent about one hour looking at the diagnostic effectiveness for these patients of the thyroid function test and at how much extra information is provided by a scan. Several of you are now better at interpreting these data'…and so on.
5. Try to isolate where general improvements are needed and list these. For example, this could be in terms of learners' ability in examining the thyroid and finding abnormalities, poor technique, or lack of knowledge. Suggestions for further reading may be appropriate.
6. Leave the session on an up-beat note. Praise the advances that the learners or trainees have made, rather than refocus on the inadequacies. If you have done your job well, the learners will have understood the rules and will act accordingly.
7. Formal teaching rounds should form part of a learning continuum either from undergraduate or postgraduate training institutions' syllabus or as part of the previously agreed contract between trainer and trainees. It is important to keep a record of each session so that progression can be seen and monitored to ensure the educational objectives are achieved over a period of time.
8. Finally, teaching episodes can become complimentary to each other, whether facilitated by the same trainer or by a group of trainers. This requires each having a knowledge of the subjects already covered. A spreadsheet of topics and teaching episodes pinned up on the wall of a clinical room provides a useful reference chart.

167

BUSINESS ROUNDS

Most of the preceding discussion on teaching rounds apply directly to the business round. However, there are some very specific business round characteristics that make it one of the most valuable learning experiences for both the trainer and the trainees.

Business rounds should involve all the staff who have a direct input into the management of patients on the ward. They provide the commonest type of ward teaching for postgraduate professional development. Maximum benefit can be gained from this useful two way process if trainees are encouraged to share knowledge derived from individual study with the group including the senior staff.

In effect, these are usually more informal than training rounds. While the numbers involved will be smaller, this may be a much more diverse group. It may include doctors, nurses and physiotherapists, all of whom may be at different levels of experience. These can range from house officer to consultant or staff nurse to ward sister.

Preparation for 'the round' is part of everyday working life in a hospital. Unlike on the training round, it is patients, their treatment and progress that are the central focus. Concentration is therefore inevitably on practice rather than theory. Conditions are discussed only in so far as they directly relate to the individual.

168

Most wards/units deal with a finite number and type of conditions so the longer staff work there the greater their specialist knowledge. This allows them to move from simple knowledge gathering and understanding to higher cognitive levels of analysis and synthesis. Here, they can readily make appropriate differential diagnoses, organise tests, discuss results and, with their combined skills, bring a holistic view to decision making, diagnoses and the formulation of a care plan. Such teaching is generally opportunistic and geared towards making decisions. At the same time, if new learning situations arise, plans can be made for formal teaching sessions around them at a later stage.

Patient consent is obviously less of an issue here than for teaching rounds. However, some ethical considerations do occur. A prime example would be when junior staff is putting into practice new skills such as insertion of a chest drain or placement of a pacemaker.

There is less chance to plan the environment apart from the normal routine of the ward. However, some adjustments can and should be made under particular circumstances such as, test results, discussion of particular lines of management or potential outcomes likely to upset patients. The way senior clinicians manage such problems is extremely important in influencing staff attitudes. Further, the patient usually knows those on the business round so particular care must be taken not to shake his or her confidence in the team looking after them. No undermining credibility with injudicious comments. Such behaviour reflects more on the person making the remarks than on those receiving them!

Ward staff have a unique opportunity to know a patient in depth. They should be encouraged to show initiative by reading about particular conditions. Instead of offering lists of findings to the senior making business rounds and expecting him or her to decide, they should attempt to solve problems themselves. The question 'So what?' after the presentation of facts is invaluable in encouraging the trainees to put their knowledge into action in the clinical situation.

The major purpose of professional training is to improve informed decision-making. Therefore, junior staff should take every opportunity to safely display their diagnostic, proposed treatment and follow-up capabilities. The outcome of clinical interventions on a disease process in an acutely ill patient provides instant feedback on the problem-solving and decision-making abilities of those involved. This provides excellent motivation to learn further, not only on the round, but also in other associated formal teaching activities such as clinical audit.

APPRAISAL AND ASSESSMENT

Over time, clinical organisation and leadership abilities can also be assessed on the ward. This gives valuable insight into interpersonal relationships not just at ward level but with staff in the laboratories, x-ray, other units and external agencies such as general practitioners. Evidence of good ethics and discipline in ward administration, keeping clinical notes, ordering relevant investigations, and following these up appropriately may be shown.

Trainees must learn to write succinct and timely discharge letters. This demonstrates clarity of thought about disease processes as applied to particular individuals, and their clinical consequences. Over a defined period of time, various ward procedures and techniques can also be taught, learned, and carried out until mastery is achieved.

169

General ward work standards culminating in business rounds allows for regular staff appraisal and assessment. At the beginning of an attachment to any ward or unit, postgraduate trainees should have time with their educational supervisor to discuss and agree their aims and objectives for the attachment period. Usually, this runs six or twelve months. At this stage, time spent aligning a particular individual's wants with what the trainer perceives their needs to be can greatly enhance teaching and learning within the unit. The protracted time period spent working alongside supervisors during an attachment facilitates attitude assessment in a way that is impossible in short courses or in single teaching episodes.

Every two to three months during an attachment, time should be devoted to one-to-one discussion between supervisor and trainee to review the latter's perception of the attachment and whether his or her objectives are being met. Alteration of these objectives or in the training process can be made by mutual agreement and reviewed in a further meeting a maximum of two months later.

At the end of the time, arrange a final meeting for the purpose of overall assessment. This should include assessing the trainee's aptitude for the particular branch of medicine and provide an opportunity for career guidance. If full and open discussions have taken place at regular intervals, there should be no surprises on either side, as to the overall outcome of the attachment.

SUMMARY

Clinical teaching can be exciting, of a high standard and personally rewarding for both teacher and learner. For this to happen the complexity of the clinical environment must be recognised and its positive attributes used to provide the best possible educational experience.

This entails:
- Involving the patient.
- Choosing clear goals that are also appropriate to the setting and patient's problems.
- Adapting those goals and teaching strategies to the existing needs, capabilities and experience of the learners.
- Using a variety of approaches designed to maintain motivation.

- These should include a high proportion of learner activities and feedback to them on their performance on these.
- Summarising at the end.

This section sets the context for the involvement of patients in medical training whether at undergraduate or postgraduate level. Most of the chapter is devoted to training at ward level, but the messages are easily adapted to teaching in general practice. Give time to preparation in order to structure the training periods. When properly used, the presence of clinical material can enliven teaching episodes, making the learning more meaningful and enjoyable, not just to the trainee but also the trainer.

CHAPTER 12
Teaching in the Theatre

MIKE WALKER & RODNEY PEYTON

INTRODUCTION

THIS CHAPTER deals with the teaching and learning of practical skills, and outlines a very powerful four stage process. This format is equally valid for teaching other skills such as taking an ECG, inserting a pacemaker or in minor surgical procedures such as tying knots or removing small skin lesions. It will be discussed primarily in the context of the operating theatre.

The concept of workmanship

The operating theatre provides a unique training environment. In many instances the trainer is dependent on the trainee's assistance meaning that they share many experiences especially during more difficult procedures.

In this one-to-one situation, the trainee can watch the trainer applying the underlying principles of his knowledge and skill base in complex practical situations. Therefore, it constitutes a classical apprenticeship with the trainer as a role model both for carrying out the procedure and handling stress. Witnessing taking decisions under pressure, and the interpersonal relationships between the surgeon as operating theatre leader and the rest of the staff, leaves a marked impression on trainees developing their surgical ethic.

Throughout their career, surgeons must continue to learn and develop. Much of this comes from reflecting on day-to-day operating theatre practice and any serious consideration of teaching and learning in surgery must take account of how surgeons learn to conceptualize and develop their work. One way of thinking about this is through the notion of 'workmanship'.

It has been suggested that there is a continuum ranging from 'the workmanship of risk' to the 'workmanship of certainty'. If we consider the use of charcoal on paper, the line once drawn can never be removed. It can be added to, blurred or disguised but once the white cartridge paper has a charcoal mark it can never be taken away. There is always the risk that the intention may not be consistently reflected in the result. In general, that is how artists work. It is the unique image thus produced that is most highly prized.

At the other end of the spectrum is 'the workmanship of certainty'. The outcome is governed as tightly as possible by jigs, precision tools and moulds so that every finished product is like the last as on an assembly line. The more freehand in the work, the more unique the finished product is liable to be.

Where is a surgeon in this spectrum? Certainly, in the early phases of training, whether it be a junior surgeon starting out in his career or a senior surgeon learning a new technique, work must be strictly governed to assure certainty and minimise risk as far as possible. Patient safety demands this approach. The concept of learning 'one safe method', from tying a surgical knot to undertaking a pneumonectomy, has been constructed to build in as many elements of certainty as possible.

The whole practice of joint replacement has flourished because its founders insisted on a rigorous, step by step process with precise measurements and special tools. Again, it was the 'measured' annuloplasty introduced by Carpentier that took mitral and tricuspid repairs from a very 'risky' business with an 'uncertain' outcome, to a reproducible operation with predictably good results.

If surgery is about building-in certainty and eliminating risk through a measured approach, then clearly surgeons, especially trainee surgeons, must acquire this general philosophy during their training. However, a purely measured scientific approach cannot be used in all situations. There are many variables related to the patients such as age and previous medical history as well as the uniqueness of a particular disease process as related to the individual.

Coupled with this are unforeseen complications during an operation which need immediate solutions. This is where surgery becomes an art form with the application of basic principles adapted by the light of experience providing the basis of sound surgical judgement. The combination of a solid training in basic techniques plus a guided apprenticeship in the employment of these techniques in a clinical situation is therefore necessary. Such a learning environment needs to be produced by those responsible for training.

THE TRAINEE

How should the training be organised? It begins with the arrival of the trainee on the surgical firm. In the first few days time must be found for an in-depth discussion on the trainee's present level of experience and competence and on what is available in the department.

Trainees should come to the meeting with a reasonable outline of what they wish to achieve over the specified time. They may need two or three days walking the wards to be able to clearly formulate their ideas. Their *wants* have to be put in the context of what the trainer perceives their *needs* to be. This is based on the trainer's previous experience of the particular trainee or other trainees at the same developmental stage on the firm.

The discussion's outcome should be realistic about whether a procedure can be learned in the time available, whether it is appropriate for that trainee, at that time in training and chosen career path. A general practice trainee on a surgical ward should not necessarily have the same training programme as a purely surgical trainee even though he or she may wish to 'have a go' at a particular technique.

173

A formal or informal learning contract is drawn up between the teacher and the learner, specifying what the teacher and/or colleagues agree to teach and, most importantly, what the learner agrees to learn in a given period of time. This provides the trainee with a set of objectives, progress towards the realization of which should be reviewed after a number of months, when further objectives or course corrections could be determined for the remaining time on the unit until the final review takes place. This review would normally consist of a viva between the trainee and the educational supervisor. It seeks to establish, firstly, factual information such as what experiences they had during the period, what operations they had observed or assisted in, what skills or procedures they had been taught, and secondly, what they had actually learned from these experiences.

This review provides the opportunity for both reflection upon and consolidation of the trainees learning, giving an opportunity to identify continuing learning needs, and also feedback to the unit with regard to their educational provision. It forms the basis of reports to the training authority or other references.

APPROACHES TO TEACHING

The next consideration is whether it is appropriate to learn skills or knowledge in the operating theatre. The trainee can be taught, and continue to practice, many basic procedures in a simulated environment so that mastery is achieved at a pace appropriate to the individual.

Activities such as tying surgical knots, bowel anastomosis, drilling and screwing bone, basic knowledge of instruments or their manipulation on a video monitor can be taught in a simulated environment leading to much more efficient use of theatre time. Surgically important anatomy, including common anomalies and complications of specific techniques can be studied in advance. Checking the knowledge base before rather than during the operation is best when the trainee is learning a new procedure. Questioning can distract the mental process and interfere with the learning of the skill.

In surgery there has been a tendency to teach operations from start to finish. It is assumed that the trainee is able to absorb everything about a prolonged procedure at one time. This can be totally counter-productive, tiring the individual and making information or skill retention much less likely.

Break down a lengthy operation into steps and consider each a separate training process. Possibly, only one step will be taught during a particular case. This prevents a one-hour operation stretching two or more and frustrating trainer, trainee, anaesthetist, and theatre nurses. As well, prolonged anaesthesia may endanger the patient.

Teaching in small increments may prolong an operation by 25-30%. Usually, this is quite long enough for the step to be well learned. When some steps are especially difficult, encouraging the trainee to carry out the whole operation in the early learning phase makes for nervousness and exhaustion. Far better that the trainer carry out the operation until he or she reaches the appropriate step, then slow down and thoroughly teach that particular step. Afterwards, the trainer finishes the operation. This leads to much greater effectiveness and efficiency in the use of theatre time. The trainee is happy because he or she learned a specific part of the procedure and the trainer knows that he or she taught it properly.

Rather like learning a piece of music, it is not necessary to go back to the beginning each time a mistake is made, but rather to repeat the appropriate few bars as often as is necessary to reach the required standard. Once all the bars are known, then the piece can be put together. The same holds true for surgery. Only when all the steps have been properly learned should the trainee attempt the operation from start to finish. Undoubtedly, surgery has its tense moments but relaxation is also necessary for all involved and unnecessary prolongation of stress by over-zealous teaching can be totally counter productive. The old concept of 'see one, do one and teach one' has no place in surgical training.

Again, the key is not to see the whole session as a training event, but rather to decide what training should take place and then to use appropriate parts of theatre time accordingly. A brief coffee room discussion prior to the case can clarify the session's objectives for one or a number of trainees. Objectives for each will be different. For instance, in the same case, a new SHO and an experienced Registrar can undertake different learning tasks such as skin suturing and the performance of a bowel resection.

THE FOUR STAGE APPROACH TO TEACHING SKILLS

This teaching method is based on the hierarchy of skills as outlined in Chapter Four. The first priority is making the trainee fully aware of the procedure and the steps involved in carrying it out. It is rather reminiscent of learning to drive a car. It may look easy, especially when done by an expert, but the reality may be somewhat different!

When the student is to have an opportunity to learn and carry out a manoeuvre in the near future, attention to detail is automatically increased. The first stage of the teaching process relies on the internal drive towards developing a new skill and does not involve any commentary. Instead, the particular skill is performed normally, in real time, and with speech limited to asking for instruments or instructing the assisting staff and anything else likely to occur during the procedure.

Therefore, by being shown the whole picture first, the trainee gets to know what is expected. Otherwise, he or she sees disjointed parts. It is like being presented with pieces of a jigsaw without being shown the picture on the box. It becomes more difficult to work out how the various individual parts fit together in a smooth procedure.

This is exaggerated by any complications and the normal process of the operation is disrupted. The trainee should have the opportunity of seeing and conceptualising the skill normally and be able to concentrate on what the surgeon is doing. This gives the trainee the general outline of the procedure, the hooks on which to base his understanding.

In the second step, the trainee comes to understand exactly what is required. The surgeon carries out the procedure, explaining it in detail. The trainee is encouraged to ask questions to clarify any issues.

In the third step, again the surgeon carries out the procedure but this time has the trainee talk through the procedure. The surgeon listens carefully at this stage, asking questions to make sure the trainee understands the sequence and key issues before undertaking the skill himself.

In the final step, surgeons allow trainees to undertake the procedure under close supervision, having them describe carefully what they are going to do at key points before the manoeuvre is carried out. These four steps benefit the trainee while ensuring patients' safety and minimising the likelihood of unintended outcomes such as perforation of a vessel, bowel, or ureter.

Moving directly from stage one to stage four is the theory behind certain game shows. In these, members of the public watch an expert carry out a procedure (for instance parcelling an awkwardly shaped object with a square piece of paper) and are then expected to carry out that procedure themselves without fully understanding how to do it. The whole show depends on it being very difficult to do and thus the participants' clumsy activities and consequent embarrassment entertains viewers. It is obvious that this is not the way to ensure the safe learning of a skill in surgery. The four-stage basic teaching process is as follows:

1. Demonstration of the normal procedure at normal speed.
2. The surgeon carries out the procedure again with full explanations and the trainee is encouraged to ask questions.
3. The surgeon performs the procedure for a third time, with the trainee describing each step and being questioned on key issues. The surgeon provides any necessary correction. This step continues until the surgeon is satisfied that the trainee fully understands the procedure.
4. The trainee now carries out the procedure under close supervision, describing each key step before it is taken.

It is vital to appreciate that learning a skill demands intense concentration. There is always a temptation for the teacher to ask questions unrelated to the skill being undertaken. These may concern complications which may arise or anatomical details irrelevant to that particular case. Even background idle chatter about another case or last night's faculty dinner may distract someone concentrating on learning a skill for the first time.

Most surgeons are well aware of instances when operations do not run to plan and they have to think about how they are going to proceed. The majority prefers silence in the theatre to help concentration at such times. They become irritated by distractions. The same physiology is present in a trainee working a new skill. The previous analogy with driving a car is also relevant here. Most can remember being told to push in the clutch, change gear, use the indicators and watch the rear view mirror at the same time as controlling the steering wheel. They remember their frustration until those procedures became second nature. Similarly, when learning a surgical skill it is all too easy for a 'surgical master' to forget how difficult it is to acquire new skills and to hinder the process by adding unnecessary distractions.

Sometimes such distractions are motivated by a genuine desire to help the trainee 'learn' everything there is to know about the procedure in one fell swoop. At others they may indicate the trainer's incipient boredom. This is less likely if a clearly defined teaching objective for a specific part of the operation is decided in advance. Throughout the rest of the procedure there is, then, ample time for discussion on other matters when the trainee does not have to concentrate so heavily on learning a skill.

Mastery in a surgical skill is achieved through the three phases of acquisition by drill, repetition and practice. It is best to teach the surgical novice one safe method for an operative procedure by drill, using the four-stage process as above. Repetition of the method in similar cases gives confidence. During this stage, the trainer's input can be slowly withdrawn first, from the table, then from the operating theatre and then from being readily available somewhere in the building. Too often in the past, trainees have been closely supervised until they seem competent and then senior support has been suddenly withdrawn. Independence should increase gradually, aiding further refinement of skills and preventing the formation of bad habits. Continued practice gives experience which can be reinforced by reading around the subject or seeing other methods of carrying out the same procedure. The skill gradually becomes semi-automatic and can be adapted to other situations.

VARIATIONS IN THE FOUR STAGE APPROACH

THE NOVICE

In practice, there are several variations of the four-stage approach. The demonstration is best carried out at the table, but specific portions of an operation may be shown on video to the same effect. It is important, however, to remember not to provide a full explanation on the first run-through. If the video has a teaching soundtrack, then it should be turned down when first showing the pertinent part, a true 'silent' demonstration. The second stage may be covered by turning up the volume and having a surgeon on hand to fully discuss the key points. This may be further assisted by the use of slides or simulator. The third stage works best in the operating theatre but can be carried out with a video, if actual operating theatre experience has been used for step one or step two. Obvious constraints inherent in using video or slides is lack of active involvement. As it is estimated that we retain 5% of what we hear, 10% of what we see but up to 90% of what we do, practical experience is clearly essential. The basic sequence is as we do, we learn and as we learn we achieve mastery.

Sometimes multiple steps can be gone through in the same operation. For instance, take suturing. Even continuous sutures can be taught by demonstrating a number of stitches in a single wound, the surgeon talking through them, the trainee talking the surgeon through some and then actually doing some themselves. This can be used as a set of individual steps in bowel anastomosis or the three ends of an aorta bi-femoral anastomosis.

EXPERIENCED STAFF

A variant of the four-stage procedure is also useful in assessing the competence of more senior trainees in carrying out specific tasks on first joining a surgical team. The first step is, as before, demonstrating the procedure in real time without any particular explanation. This is followed by a full discussion with the senior trainee as to whether the technique demonstrated is precisely the technique they have employed in the past and are comfortable with. If not, any differences should be highlighted. If the consultant or the trainee perceives these as significant they should be taught using the three remaining stages. On the other hand, if the trainee indicates familiarity with the technique the trainer can move directly to the fourth step wherein the trainee carries out the procedure, explaining what is about to be done beforehand. This allows the trainer to assess the trainee's knowledge, skill base, and competence and determine whether further supervision is necessary.

For senior trainees joining a unit, therefore, the stages are as follows:

1. Demonstration at normal speed.
2. Discussion with the trainee, highlighting any differences in technique.
3a. If there are no apparent significant differences, trainee carries out the procedure under guidance.
3b. If there are significant differences, then stages two, three and four in a normal four-stage procedure should be undertaken.

THE SIGNIFICANCE OF FEEDBACK

The significance and importance of feedback is discussed in Chapter Three on motivation in adult learning. It is stressed that feedback provides a source of motivation as well as information essential to adjusting and improving efforts. In order to function in this way feedback has to be positive.

Traditionally in medical education, most comments on trainee performance stress what went badly, or where they went wrong. Having been brought up in that method, most trainees when asked to discuss their performance will begin with a list of mistakes, missed opportunities and general condemnation of their own efforts. Undoubtedly, some trainers feel analysing a performance and pinpointing mistakes helps to boost their own ego by confirming their expert status. This sort of criticism has little to do with helping the learner's motivation.

Learners often have a good idea of what went wrong and only need help where they have not recognised a mistake or are unclear how to avoid it. However, it must be stressed, that important issues must be aired and that if the trainee does not bring out major points when the conversation is directed towards them, the trainer has a responsibility to clearly address such concerns.

Therefore, having watched trainees' efforts with a particular procedure, the trainer should ask what they felt went well or what they were particularly happy with. A number of surgeons on first thinking about this particular style of questioning feel it superfluous and unnecessary. Most emphatically, it is not. In the first instance, it allows the trainee to identify good practice. This can then be reinforced. Also, it allows the trainer to hear whether the trainee has insight into any problems that may have arisen. While the trainee may declare his or her happiness with incision or anastomosis, the trainer knows they were not up to standard. Active listening gives vital insight into the trainee's ability to analyze his own performance.

The trainer must then ascertain what lessons the trainee has learned and how performance might be modified or improved. At what stage of the procedure did he feel particularly uncomfortable and why? It is most important that trainees focus and reflect on improving their performance and not simply list potential bad points. Develop a positive action plan to improve practice; take decisions on implementing the next case or if, for instance hand-eye co-ordination is a problem, whether practice on a simulator may be more appropriate.

During this reflective phase, it is useful for the trainer to think over the four-stage teaching procedure in order to diagnose any problems the trainee may have. If the skill was carried out improperly, was it because the trainee had a problem with his co-ordination on instrument handling, or was the problem with his knowledge base on how to proceed? The trainer could suggest stepping back a stage, carrying out the next procedure himself and asking the trainee to describe key points in detail as the operation proceeds. It may even be necessary to step back to stage two, and for the trainer to undertake the procedure, describing and explaining each of the stages very carefully until the trainee fully grasps the concepts.

The necessity for a quiet room in theatre where the teacher and trainee or trainees can sit down to talk about cases is readily apparent. Prior to the operation, discuss clinical findings and x-rays and clearly set out each individual's objectives during the procedure. With a group of trainees it is good to decide at this time what part of the procedure is appropriate for which trainee. Structure the operation so each gets the appropriate training but recognise, for the sake of theatre staff, that it is unwise to do too much teaching on any one case. The teacher's skill is in deciding how much is too much. The teacher must remember the trainee's learning capacity and the stress level and general fatigue the teacher suffers on the job, not to mention the ability of the rest of the staff to manage changes in the list.

Nothing is more frustrating for an anaesthetist then to expect a particular operation to last an hour and then to find it dragging on two or more hours. On the other hand, it is not unknown for a frustrated surgeon to suddenly decide to finish the case quickly himself, leaving the anaesthetist to spend the next half-hour waking up a patient to whom he has just given a long-term muscle relaxant. Courtesy and co-operation go a long way and the way the surgeon treats other staff is not lost on those he is teaching.

BEYOND THE ACQUISITION OF SKILLS— ASSESSMENT AND DEVELOPMENT

Assessment in the affective domain is vital in surgical training. It is best undertaken by long term observation and discussion. There are three basic competencies related to a skill. These are the ability to carry it out, the development of competence and the standard of performance when the trainee practices independently. The innate ability to carry out a surgical procedure and the development of competence in that procedure are usually assessed in a controlled environment where the trainer is present. Certainly, no one should be allowed to carry out an operative task unaided unless they previously clearly demonstrated the ability and competence to do so.

However, performance is what trainees do when the trainer is not present. It very much depends on their attitude towards the patient, the field of surgery in general and the particular technique they have been taught. If they do not demonstrate a sense of value for that technique they may alter it or take short cuts when not being supervised.

This is not necessarily a bad thing since they may see many different operating techniques while in training and make up their own minds, on the basis of experience, which one best suits them and their patient. On the other hand, short cuts may be to the patient's detriment and fall below acceptable standards. A trainee's value system is extremely important if their performance is to match their competence. None is better positioned to assess than the trainer who spends time in close association with the trainee on the wards, in outpatients or in theatre. Surgical trainers need to be quite clear that this is an important part of their role. Since it can only be assessed by observation and discussion, they must make time to spend with their trainees, actively listening to their thoughts and aspirations, watching them as they become more senior and assessing their aptitude for leadership amongst their peers and other staff with whom they come in contact. Not only their surgical performance can be assessed, but also a more general overview of their medical ethic. Only those who spend time in the work environment with the trainee have a chance to assess this vital area and consultant supervisors must undertake this task.

Finally, the outcome of a surgical episode may not be known for days, weeks, or even months. Therefore, assessing theatre skills requires, in many cases, a long-term follow-up. While the use of log books to record operative procedures may provide some idea of the level of experience in terms of the amount and type of procedures carried out, it is totally inadequate when measuring outcomes.

The surgical audit is an integral part of the feedback chain and trainees should be encouraged to review their own patients with senior staff over the weeks or months following the surgical procedure. This can be problematical since there is a tendency not to review 'routine cases' once they have left hospital. Day cases are a particular case in point as follow up is frequently by the GP or district nurse who would be expected to deal with minor complications such as localised infections. Other complications, such as recurrence of a hernia, may not be noted for many months by which time the trainee has moved on from the unit and the case is simply referred back to the consultant involved.

It is important that trainees be given the opportunity to record and reflect on any problems developing in cases in which they have been involved. Procedures, such as sending them copies of follow-up reports, that allow this should be in place. Equally, it is important that they know what went well and, thus, reviewing only those cases with complications is inclined to give the wrong impression. Proper review of all cases is important both for the trainer and the trainee. It should not be downgraded because of service commitments or financial constraints.

PUTTING THIS CHAPTER INTO ACTION

Teaching and learning in the operating theatre provides an unparalleled opportunity for trainer and trainee to work together and learn from each other. The process begins when the trainee arrives in the unit. Time should be taken to develop an appropriate training program which can then be reviewed and refined if necessary over the succeeding months. Once the objectives have been set then their appropriateness to training in the theatre setting should be scrutinised.

The teaching of a skill follows a basic four-stage process. The stages may be supplemented or replaced, in part, by the use of videos and slides.

1. Demonstration in real time.
2. Trainer performs with full discussion and trainee asks questions.
3. Trainer performs and asks questions with trainee talking through and discussing the procedure until the key areas are fully understood.
4. Trainee performs the procedure, describing any key areas before carrying them out.

Following as soon as possible after the procedure, a critique should determine what the trainee feels went well and points for improvement. The trainer can diagnose any problems, primarily deciding whether any are concerned with hand/eye co-ordination or with basic understanding of the technique. The former may be addressed by training in a simulated environment, and the latter, by reverting to an earlier level of the four-stage process.

For senior trainees, the four-stage procedure can be slightly modified to determine their levels of expertise and it becomes:

1. Demonstration in real time with no particular explanations.
2. Discussion with the trainee, highlighting any areas of departure from previous training.
3. Decision is then made as to whether to follow steps 2, 3 and 4 of the four-stage procedure or, if there are no apparent significant differences, proceed straight to stage 4 whereby the trainee carries out the procedure, discussing key areas with the trainer as he or she does so.

Note the importance of attitude, the vital ingredient in turning a level of competence into a standard of continuing performance. This is crucial in any professional development and it is incumbent on the trainer to develop a close working relationship with the trainee, building rapport in order to be in a position to make such assessments.

Finally, beware fatigue. Periods of instruction in theatre can be very intense, the more so if personnel have had long periods on call, lack of sleep, been involved in a tedious outpatient session or have other distractions disturbing their concentration either within or outside the hospital. Whether it is the trainee or trainer who is tired, training should be stopped.

CHAPTER 13
Education in the Outpatient Clinic: Purposes, Content and Methods

COLIN COLES

INTRODUCTION

THIS CHAPTER explores learning in the outpatient setting. It looks at teachers' and learners' roles in this context and considers other ways of teaching besides seeing actual patients. A consistent theme running through the chapter is that the teacher's role is to help trainees learn.

Outpatient clinics are an essential part of any hospital service. Medical staff sees patients either to diagnose clinical problems or to follow up their management. Patients are likely to be seen in an office setting rather than a ward, possibly with trainees or students present, and frequently in the presence of other clinical staff such as nurses. Increasingly, outpatient clinics are held at smaller local hospitals, in outreach clinics in general practices and health centres where the consultant travels to the patient rather than vice versa.

Undoubtedly, the outpatient clinic provides a very valuable educational environment for trainees. However, the pressure on service work, such as seeing a large volume of patients in a rather short space of time, severely limits the teaching and learning that takes place. Education is largely opportunistic in this setting. Teachers must teach and trainees must learn whatever is possible from patients being seen at that particular time. Planned education, in the sense of 'covering the syllabus', is much more difficult, as one cannot predict the patients that will be seen.

Nevertheless, there is an enormous potential for good education in the outpatient clinic. So how can this best be achieved? What is the content of outpatient clinic teaching and what methods are there for achieving effective learning?

CONTENT

The specific content of education in an outpatient clinic depends on the speciality involved. However, two general aspects of outpatient clinic education apply to all specialities. The first is for trainees to understand how to make a diagnosis and communicate this to patients. The second is to understand how to develop professional judgement.

Diagnosing is a crucial role for the clinician in an outpatient clinic. A general practitioner refers the majority of patients and some diagnostic screening has already taken place. Some clinical examinations and tests may already have been carried out. The hospital clinician might have been asked to confirm the general practitioner's opinion, or the patient might have been referred because the diagnosis is as yet unknown.

The nature of clinical diagnosis has been well researched. It is generally accepted that the diagnostic process is one of problem solving, probably involving some hypothesis testing, and requiring further clinical tests and investigations on this and some other occasion. Trainees need to learn how to make diagnoses, what clinical indications to seek out, and what possible alternative or additional diagnoses there might be.

The next phase is telling the patient the diagnosis and its likely management. Frequently, the patient is anxious and bad news might need to be conveyed. At the very least, a patient's understanding of his or her problem and its management can greatly influence their compliance. The nature of this difficult communication process and the breaking of bad news have also been well researched. The findings indicate that professional practice is deficient and far from satisfactory in this area.

The way diagnoses are most commonly made and communicated in an outpatient clinic has been described as 'doctor-centred' or 'the medical model'. The doctor asks patients questions, proceeds to tell them what is wrong and what needs to be done. No doubt, this model is efficient in terms of time but its effectiveness has been challenged. It can lead to inappropriate and missed diagnoses since the doctor is pursuing a specific line of enquiry which might ignore other possibilities. Moreover, doctor-centred interviewing does not help patients understand their problems and their implications.

An alternative approach that addresses such problems is 'patient-centred' interviewing. This is particularly valuable when the patient has a chronic or long standing condition and where a high level of patient compliance is necessary for satisfactory clinical management. Such instances might be encountered when dealing with diabetes, asthma and renal failure. These patients have a large degree of clinical responsibility and autonomy, and so an understanding of the conditions and their role in the maintenance of their health is crucial. Doctors can influence clinical management not only by competent medical care, but also by shaping how patients feel about the disease, their sense of commitment to the treatment and their ability to control and contain its impact on their lives.

Patient-centred interviewing entails a more open and two-way conversation so that the patient, as well as the clinician, understands the condition. This form of interviewing gathers appropriate information enabling the doctor to arrive at the diagnosis and explores the patient's health beliefs. The assumptions patients make about their symptoms, the condition itself, their knowledge and understanding of disease process all greatly influence how (and even whether) the patient will comply with the prescribed management.

183

Problems arise because many trainees have never experienced (let alone been taught about) patient-centred interviewing. Research suggests it is uncommon in general medical practice but then 'diagnosing' or 'communication to patients' is seldom formally taught but is largely 'picked up' through some form of osmosis. Needless to say, poor practice may well be picked up in the same manner. Teaching in the outpatient clinic should address both of these issues.

The second use of content in outpatient clinic education is for trainees to learn to make professional judgements. Again, it is unusual for trainees to be taught this fundamental feature of a consultant's professional practice.

Schon observed that much professional work occurs in what he describes as the 'swampy lowlands' of practice. Most professional problems do not have neat, simple solutions but are 'messy'. A key professional attribute is the ability to make judgements in unpredictable situations. The professional must be prepared for the unexpected.

What then is teaching *content* when it comes to educating trainees about professional judgement? Formal theory, or 'propositional knowledge', is found in written form - books, journals, articles and such. It is the basis of most formal teaching. Personal theory is one's practical knowledge or know how, acquired through experience. Both kinds of theory influence one's professional judgements through a somewhat complex interaction.

We are exposed to formal theory, we are taught it, and we learn it. We even pass examinations in it. But it does not directly influence our professional judgement. We do not 'apply' theory to practice. Rather, we transform and interpret formal theory, and incorporate it into our practice.

Our personal theory - what we believe, assume and value - helps us make sense of our world, and hence our professional practice. It forms a basis for our professional actions and judgements. It informs and directs what we do. We create our own personal knowledge. No two people have the same personal knowledge. Even people with similar experiences will have a different personal knowledge.

Therefore, we create or construct our personal theory over time as a result of who we are, what we have experienced, how we have interpreted those experiences, and through our very personal transformation of formal knowledge. Little wonder then, that teaching professional judgement is so difficult!

There is a further problem. Our personal theories comprise not just with what we believe we do (our espoused theory) but also our theory-in-use (what we actually do). The two theories can be different. We may say we believe something but in reality our actions suggest a quite different theoretical basis. Clearly, this lack of insight into the nature of our personal theory can cause problems in professional practice and teaching.

It is commonly believed there is a theory-practice gap: that what people know in theory, is distinct from what they actually do in practice. Much is known in theory but people do not use that knowledge in practice. However plausible this view, it is overly simplistic. In reality, there is a theory-theory gap, or, more particularly, series of gaps. There is a gap between formal theory and personal theory. It is our personal, rather than formal, theory that determines our practice. We need to recreate the formal theory in our own context so that it can be incorporated into a personal theory that can inform our practice. Any gap between our espoused theory and our theory-in-use is allowable so long as we know that it exists.

Teaching professional judgement has been seriously neglected. Again, it is acquired through osmosis. However, we now know much about its nature and importance, and it should become a central feature of postgraduate education. The outpatient clinic is an ideal location for achieving this.

METHODS

This discussion of content for outpatient clinic education has highlighted two broad areas common to all specialities - the need for trainees to learn how to diagnose and communicate a diagnosis to patients, and a need to learn how to develop one's professional judgement. The important educational principle for medical teachers to grasp is that these develop through an interaction between what trainees do in the practice setting and what they study in relation to their practice, in other words when they relate theory and practice.

Before looking more closely at methods for outpatient clinic education, it is important to reiterate two general principles (developed further in other chapters in this book) concerning the nature of teaching and learning:

- The teacher's main function is to establish and maintain a positive learning environment. There must be an atmosphere of trust, openness and honesty between the teacher and the learner. The teacher should be a 'critical friend' able to provide the learner with support and constructive feedback on his or her performance. An effective teacher should be capable of self reflection on his or her own practice, and offer learners opportunities for reflection on theirs, that is to provide a mirror to learners' practice so they see themselves as others see them.

- Learners should see themselves as professional self-educators, that is, as active participants directing their own education, and so should make best use of their time. This will mean resolving the inevitable tensions between education and service work. They should see their role as one of 'elaborating' their knowledge, that is making links and connections between their experiences, their reading and their thinking. They should develop ways of 'capturing the learning' from their everyday clinical experience.

A MODEL FOR OUTPATIENT CLINIC EDUCATION

The following four-phase model can guide education in the outpatient setting:

1. A clinician (preferably the trainee's supervisor) demonstrates some clinical practice, which the trainee observes and then discusses with the clinician.

2. The trainee reflects on these observations and discussions, and 'captures the learning' through reading and writing.

3. The trainee practices while being supervised by the clinician who gives constructive feedback on the trainee's performance.

4. The trainee performs unsupervised, though with continuing support, and has opportunities to discuss his or her performance with the supervisor.

185

These four phases of outpatient education will now be described more fully using as an illustration how to teach trainees about breaking bad news.

Demonstration and Discussion

During this first phase, a trainee observes his or her supervisor breaking bad news in the everyday setting of an outpatient clinic. At a suitable moment, as soon as possible afterwards in a spirit of enquiry and development, they debrief on the supervisor's performance. The supervisor should be open in reviewing his or her own performance, and describe personal theory concerning the breaking of bad news. This should involve not only what he or she knows (formal knowledge) about breaking bad news but also what he or she *knows about* when it comes to breaking bad news (personal knowledge). Crucially, the supervisor should identify moments within the demonstration where judgements and critical decisions about how to proceed, what line to take, what not to do were made.

This debriefing should lead to a more general discussion about breaking bad news, generalising from the particular incident observed to establish criteria and principles for action.

This first phase should be repeated more than once, with trainees building up an increasingly complex picture of the way bad news is handled. They may have the opportunity to watch other clinicians. They should have ample opportunity to explore their own thinking through discussions with their supervisor.

Reflection

As a result of observing the supervisor's demonstration of breaking bad news, the trainee should undertake a period of reflection in order to 'capture' and to consolidate his or her own learning about this topic. Such reflection is likely to require private study. The student will need to read around the subject, thinking about the issues, identifying his or her own personal theory, making sense of what is being read, incorporating the formal knowledge into personal knowledge, and writing notes to consolidate the learning and to provide a basis for subsequent discussions with the supervisor. It is important that supervisors should be able to recommend appropriate literature. They do not need to have at their finger tips a reading list for every topic but they do need to encourage trainees to use various information sources (such as libraries). The important role of the supervisor is to encourage reflection and reading. This should lead to further discussions with the supervisor (and others) on this topic, perhaps during routine supervision sessions.

It is crucial for both the trainee and the supervisor to value this reflection. It is not enough to merely observe a procedure or even worse to carry out the procedure without any instruction at all. It is essential trainees learn from experience, and this requires time to be set aside from routine clinical work to enable reflection to occur.

Performing Under Supervision and Debriefing

The third phase is for the trainee to break bad news in an outpatient clinic under the clinician's supervision when both agree the time is ready. The function of supervision at this stage is twofold; first so the supervisor can ensure that both the patient's and relatives' needs are met. Secondly, the supervisor has to carry out a debriefing with the trainee.

This should occur as soon as possible after the event. It is important that the supervisor help the trainee describe his or her personal theory of breaking bad news, and relate it to what actually happened.

The debrief is likely to raise wide-ranging issues of bad news breaking, and possibly lead to discussion of the trainee's performance in other areas. The trainee will need support because of the stressful nature of breaking bad news. It is an emotionally charged and sensitive situation for all concerned.

This phase should occur more than once. In between, the trainee should be encouraged to observe further demonstrations by experienced clinicians and to reflect, read, discuss, and capture the learning for him or herself.

Performing Unsupervised

The trainee and supervisor must now agree when the trainee is ready to perform this procedure unsupervised. Discussion might involve other members of the clinical team, including nurses. However, the supervisor's responsibility has not ended. Unsupervised performance should also be analysed. Clearly, the supervisor will not have observed the performance, and the debriefing will rely on the trainee's description. As with the third phase, this is likely to lead to a wider discussion of breaking bad news, and to require personal support.

This phase would be incomplete without it being repeated until the trainee and the supervisor agree the trainee is confident enough to break bad news routinely. Having said this, it is likely that the trainee (and indeed the supervisor) may want to discuss occasions where breaking bad news did not go routinely or where they require personal support following a difficult experience.

Discussion of This Example

This example of outpatient education and the model on which it is based highlights a number of general principles:

—An essential prerequisite for high quality education is a safe climate within which trainees can learn. This requires supervisors and trainees to be open and honest concerning their performance of clinical procedures.

—Outpatient education must be deliberate and monitored despite its opportunistic nature. It is important for trainees to capture the learning through discussion, reflection, reading and writing. Educational supervisors and trainees should keep records of the phases of development reached in the learning of particular clinical procedures.

—The interrelationship between the phases is as important as the phases themselves. The phases are sequential but they are not linear. Rather, they represent cycles of development. Each phase leads on to the next. However, there should be continual reiteration between them.

187

—Dealing with trainees' emotional reactions while performing sensitive clinical procedures, such as breaking bad news, should become a routine part of the educational process. It is very important that supervisors recognise the need for personal support and, possibly, trainee counselling. They must feel confident to provide this.

Debriefing and Constructive Feedback
At all stages, there is a need for debriefing based on providing constructive feedback. A scheme for this is as follows:

1. Observe or describe the performance.
2. Identify what went well (trainee first, then supervisor).
3. Identify what did not go well (trainee first, then supervisor).
4. What does the trainee want to improve?
5. What does the supervisor consider the trainee needs to improve?
6. Agree some learning goals.
7. Carry out the recovery education to achieve these goals.
8. Review progress and learning outcomes.
9. Set new learning goals.

—Debriefing begins with the trainee describing what he or she believes went well in a procedure the supervisor has observed. The supervisor (and anyone else) then adds positive comments. There are two reasons for beginning positively; first, it establishes good practice criteria (and noting that some are already present in the trainee's actions). Second, and equally important, it provides a constructive atmosphere within which to deal with any problems or difficulties. Many trainees say that they never know how well they are doing, only how badly. They are rarely given positive comments.

—The trainee next says what did not go well in that piece of practice. Here, the supervisor's role is to encourage trainees to explore their actions as fully as possible, in effect, to see themselves as others see them. It is important for trainees to develop insight. Supervisors find that most can criticise themselves, and this avoids the often difficult task of pointing out their faults. Once the trainee has listed what he or she sees as weaknesses, the supervisor (and any others) can then add what they saw as negative aspects.

—The trainee then reviews the positive and negative aspects of practice already identified (this can be helped by writing points down). This establishes their learning *wants*. These represent what trainees feel they want to learn so as to perform this piece of practice better. It is the trainee's agenda. Again, it is an important capacity for learners to develop. Without it, self-directed learning is impossible.

The supervisor next says what he or she believes are the trainee's *needs*. Although the supervisor believes these aspects of learning should be addressed for more effective practice, the trainee has not yet identified them. It is the supervisor's agenda for the trainee.

—Discussion of these two agendas, the trainee's wants and needs, provides clarification and leads to an agreed list of learning objectives, an educational plan. Priority is assigned to the more important items. Negotiation is important. Trainees will only successfully learn what they come to believe is important for them. Their learning *needs* must be transformed into their learning *wants*. Negotiation suggests mutual agreement, not the imposition of one person's agenda. Supervisors cannot make trainees learn what they do not want to learn.

—The learning agenda should then be addressed. An educational plan that is agreed in this manner becomes the basis for the trainee's self-directed learning. He or she now knows what should happen next. The supervisor's main contribution has been to help the trainee establish this plan.

—Subsequently the trainee can describe what educational activity has been undertaken to achieve the plan, and summarise his or her learning outcomes. This will lead to further discussion, and the supervisor will be able to clarify any misunderstandings or, where appropriate, add new knowledge.

—Finally, the supervisor might comment on the trainee's achievement, recalling positive elements of his or her practice identified at the outset, and thus praise achievements and indicate areas for further study.

In outpatient education this debriefing is likely to be most valuable outside clinic time and in a setting conducive to uninterrupted discussion. Shortened versions might be useful if a trainee has been observed performing come clinical activity. The first two stages (what went well and not so well) should be undertaken as soon as possible, with the remaining stages being carried forward to a more opportune moment.

Outpatient sessions with trainees should, then, allow time for educational discussions, both during and after the clinic. Inevitably, this will mean that fewer patients will be seen when a trainee is present, and adjustments to clinic routines will have to be made. Other clinic staff and hospital managers should acknowledge this. Supervisors' educational responsibilities should feature in their job plans and employment contracts.

OTHER TEACHING METHODS

So far, we have considered education in the outpatient clinic in 'real time' with 'real patients'. This is not always possible or desirable. The supervisor and trainee may have difficulty in being in the same place at the same time, and the presence of trainees might be undesirable from the viewpoint of either the patient or the clinician. Three alternatives to this are recording, simulation, and case study.

Recording

Video (and audio) recording are extremely valuable for observing clinical procedures in outpatient clinic education. In general practice, this technique has been used for many years. Recording replaced observation and provided a source for teaching unsupervised performance (such as in the fourth phase described earlier). It has several advantages over real time observations:

- It allows more economical usage of supervisors' and the trainees' time.
- It provides observation of clinical procedures that occur occasionally or out of hours.
- It allows an opportunity to check the accuracy of an observation, or to perform a deeper and more time-consuming post performance analysis.
- It allows one to see change in performance over time.

Recording also has some disadvantages.

—Being recorded can be intimidating.

—People might perform differently in the presence of recording equipment.

—Need to preserve confidentiality and obtain patient consent.

—Technical issues can cause problems. Cameras should be pointed away from windows. Microphones should be as close as possible to the people being recorded.

On balance, the strengths outweigh the weaknesses, particularly regarding convenience. Research shows being recorded does not affect clinicians. They soon adjust to the camera's presence and work the same as when unrecorded.

Audio recording can overcome some of the disadvantages of video. Technically, it is easier to arrange and one can obtain good quality sound that is important if details of the conversation need to be studied. However, it does not allow observation of people's non-verbal behaviour, which might be important from an educational standpoint.

Simulation

Simulation avoids using real patients and two approaches are common. Use of actors (or standardised patients) and role-playing.

ACTOR PATIENTS

The use of actor patients has a number of advantages:

- To control distractions in real life clinical situations.
- To focus on important clinical variables.
- To look in detail at specific aspects of a clinical procedure or particular work being undertaken in clinic.

- To lower risks to patients (though it must be recognised that actors can experience some of the same discomforts facing patients).
- To allow practice of clinical procedures at a convenient time for both supervisor and trainee.
- To truncate time (by speeding up a procedure or missing out stages).
- To repeat the practice of procedures.
- To obtain informed feedback from the actors about the clinicians' performance.

There are a number of disadvantages:

—It is difficult (or even impossible) to stimulate certain clinical conditions.
—The need to train and prepare actors thoroughly.
—The cost of employing actors.
—The need for all concerned to 'suspend their disbelief'.

ROLE PLAYING

Simulation is an alternative form of role-playing. Here, professionals are asked to adopt the role of patient with a particular condition or someone in a different profession.

The advantages of role-play are the same as for actor patients. However, professional people have the opportunity to experience something different from their normal life. The disadvantages are also similar. The main one being the difficulty of suspending one's disbelief in role play. Often clinicians feel uncomfortable in these situations, believing it to be useless 'play acting'. However, greater familiarity with actor patients and the experience of role-play, and a firm commitment to the importance of learning through experience can make this technique more acceptable and potentially useful. Role-play can be enhanced by providing accurate, detailed, and above all, relevant scenarios.

Case Study

Case study is a third alternative to learning from actual clinical experience. It provides an opportunity for clinicians, through a verbal presentation to consider, reveal and highlight essential aspects of their practice. The patient is presented abstractly, often in written form. Ideally, case studies should be based on actual cases. Clinic pathological conferences and grand rounds are common examples. Biography and autobiography patients are examples from a wider literature. Personal view columns in medical journals often provide valuable insight into illness experienced by health professionals and can become useful educational material.

Case studies have a number of advantages:

- To observe a patient through verbal description.
- To truncate time.
- To consolidate events.
- To select and focus on particular aspects of clinical practice.
- To allow wide dissemination.

There are also some disadvantages:

—Visual observation not possible.

—Misses unreported aspects of a situation.

—The purpose of the activity will constrain what is reported (for example, a clinico-pathological conference will most likely only report 'scientific' information).

—The describer's viewpoint is likely to reflect bias.

—Tendency to be overly abstract to be academic and more focused on

—theoretical aspects of a case than on clinical practice itself.

—Likely to ignore (or fail to identify) the practitioner's theories of practice.

—Less helpful educationally for those early in their career who lack concrete experience to relate to a case study.

A form of case study is 'critical incident analysis', where some aspect of practice is selected for detailed study. Particularly useful are situations that do not conform to everyday practice, as well as those that involve a unique response on the part of the practitioner, such as when a professional judgement has to be made.

Critical incident analysis is essentially self-directed. It begins with the practitioner's description of the incident, that is what led up to it, and what happened afterwards. Then, the practitioner explores his or her 'theories of practice' and considers how these differ from those that he or she considers 'espoused theories'.

Critical incident analysis is best carried out through discussion with a colleague, mentor or critical friend. It also involves writing a record of one's thoughts and ideas and allows one the opportunity of reviewing them subsequently. Indeed, revisiting the incident through a process of reflection and articulating one's thoughts, is an important feature of critical analysis, and goes with the further recording of these new thoughts in writing.

The main purpose of critical incident analysis is practitioner self-development through insights into one's own professional practice and its theoretical basis. Discussions with a supervisor or colleague can put this into a wider educational context, and further work can involve reading and writing. This approach has also been described as 'practitioner research'. Very different from conventional research, it shares its outcomes through wider dissemination in journals and may be valuable.

CONCLUSIONS

This chapter has looked at opportunities for education in outpatient clinics. It emphasised the importance of teaching the process of diagnosing and developing professional judgement. It described a four-phase method using the breaking of bad news as an example. Debriefing by constructive feedback with trainees is essential to education in this setting.

A constant theme has been seeing education from the trainee's point of view, in effect, what it means to learn something rather than to teach it. The challenge for supervisors is to unlearn what they know at present and to put themselves in the trainee's position.

Very importantly, outpatient education should be monitored and deliberate, not haphazard as it so often is at present. This is not to deny that much good education is opportunistic - teaching and learning as and when things arise. Rather, supervisors and trainees should know where they are 'in the educational process'. Supervisors should keep more notes of their trainee's progress than many do at present, and trainees need to capturing the learning from their experiences.

Outpatient clinics provide an ideal setting within which to learn. Of course, they have an even more important function in health care. Crucially, there is a need to resolve the tensions that undoubtedly exist between providing an effective clinical service and the educational needs of the professionals involved in providing it. This is the most pressing challenge at the present time.

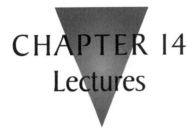

CHAPTER 14
Lectures

DUNCAN HARRIS

INTRODUCTION

HAVE YOU BEEN to lectures when you cannot remember much about the content, but a lot about the presentation or the lecturer? Here are a few examples:

- The lecturer who rambles on for an hour and who may well know what he or she is talking about, but cannot give you the slightest idea.
- The lecturer who has a magnificent set of slides changing about every 30 seconds, whilst you sit in complete darkness and feel like going to sleep; of course, you cannot note the important points because it is too dark.
- The lecturer who has many anecdotes and cases that are poured out at great length, unconnected to any theme other than showing how much experience he or she has.

- The magnificent performance with many good jokes, many superb slides of cases or of text. You remember the lecturer and the slides, but what was the lecture about?
- The most effective lectures for you probably had the following characteristics:
  —You wanted to know about the content.
  —The content was related to your experience.
  —The content had potential for your future work (or upcoming examination!)
  —The lecture was well organised.
  —The lecturer was enthusiastic.

WHY GIVE A LECTURE?

Some of the origins of lectures go back to the ancient universities. Back then there were acknowledged experts who normally only came into contact with their own designated tutees. To enable more students to hear the expert, special sessions were arranged. These sessions were rather like sermons in a church hence the derivation of the word, from lectern. The audience was there because they wished to be there.

Current time and finance pressures mean lectures take up an ever increasing proportion of teaching time. Clearly, this enables more students to be taught at the same time, so saving the need for so many lecturers. The real purpose should be to provide up-to-date information and ideas that are not easily accessible in texts or papers, or to explain or elaborate upon difficult concepts and ideas and how these should be addressed.

Unfortunately, the way lectures are organised are often quite alien to the needs of adult learners. Adult learners have the following basic needs (see Chapter Two):

- Active involvement.
- Meaningful for their needs.
- An experience based approach (both theirs and the lecturers).
- Feedback provided to the learner.
- Opportunity to reflect on the experience.
- Learning capacity addressed.

A brief consideration of each of these aspects as they apply to the giving of lectures will form the basis for the remaining sections. Active involvement seems impossible in the conventional lecture. However, with questions, small buzz groups of learners discussing a question or problem in order to come to a decision and reflection on notes there is potential for involvement. The totally theoretical lecture with no connection to anything that the learner perceives as making sense, clearly must be changed to enable the content to be more relevant and meaningful. The use of the lecturer's and the learners' experiences are usually possible and assists motivation. Feedback is difficult in a lecture but not totally impossible. Again, the use of questions, even rhetorical ones, and buzz groups can help. The same activities can be used to enable reflection. 'Learning capacity' obviously relates to learners' abilities, but there is another important facet; the amount of time that concentration is expected. To enable maximum learning efficiency, there should be 15 minute sections with a different activity. Shorter times will be appropriate if the subject is very detailed, if there is a lot of new material, if the learners are tired and if it is after lunch! The teacher's dynamism in terms of voice patterns and body language is another important cause of varying attention spans.

Clearly, what has been regarded as a conventional lecture with lots of talk by one person for an hour with no break, conflicts with all known principles of education. The dictionary definition of a lecture will not fit with the suggestions for the teaching sessions that the remainder of the chapter discusses. The intention is to change activities and use short sections. There are even some potential opportunities for micro-sleeps when the learner can switch off for a short time, but only when the lecturer wants!

195

HOW SHOULD A LECTURE BE ORGANISED?

The approach depends on the group size. For all group sizes there will be suggestions to meet the criteria for adult learners. The use of sections of 15 minutes or less and the use of activities will be incorporated for all group sizes.

The smaller group sizes are the easiest to organise for involvement, so these will be considered first. For convenience, the group sizes will be considered as:

- Less than 50.
- 50-100
- Over 100.

For all these group sizes the basic framework is the same. We will use the terms *set*, *dialogue* and *closure* to describe a lecture's three basic elements. These elements enable the preparation to be carried out in a systematic way.

SET

The analogy is rather like a theatre set. The analogy is relevant because any teacher needs to include some element of acting in their performance, especially with larger groups. There are two main considerations, the lecture environment and objectives.

The obvious part of the set will be the stage, lighting, blackout, heating and ventilation. For convenience, we will call these the environment. It may be possible to adjust the seating arrangement for smaller groups, so this would also become part of the environment. Clearly, the lecturer must be as familiar as possible with the environment: Where are the switches? What do they operate? Is it possible to have dimmed or partial lighting?

Active involvement during the lecture may be unexpected in view of learners' previous experience. Therefore, it is necessary to identify their changing roles in the parts of the lecture where such activities will occur. In addition, are you the lecturer willing to be interrupted to answer questions? Learners need to know your role too. It may be possible to identify it by your position. Standing behind a lectern makes it clear that you want no interruptions and that learners are expected to take the role of blotting paper. If you are near them in the front you have identified a different, clearly more interactive, role for yourself.

Finally, it is important from the beginning, for learners to know what the lecture is about and how it is organised so that they can make sense of it. There must be a clear identification of the purpose. The identification may be in the form of statements, sometimes called 'objectives'. These are questions that the lecture will attempt to answer or at least outline.

DIALOGUE

The dialogue is the meat of the lecture. It can be a monologue, a dialogue between the lecturer and the learners (implying that they have something to say and/or do), or a dialogue between learners (for example in buzz groups). A well-organised lecture should include two or all three variations. Remember, the whole process of teaching is about enabling learning and the learning is done by the learners not the lecturer. The content must be accurate, valid, and up-to-date. What the lecturer says or does is of no significance if learners do not learn.

CLOSURE

In a lecture where the lecturer is without a separate chairperson, ordering the end of the lecture is important.

The first step is to ask if there are any problems or questions. If there are general problems, re-iterate key issues or return to them in a future session. Other issues may be raised and their relevance to the whole group must be assessed if dealing with them is liable to take time. Some may be dealt with by suggesting that the interested person discuss them with you at a specified time. Other questions may be sufficiently important to understanding the session that a small amount of time must be spent on them.

The next step is summarising the whole lecture. The summary contains the key issues, including those arising during question time.

The final step is very short but crucial. It deals with the termination. The clear signal that the lecture has finished. The termination may be simple such as, 'there is now a break for coffee/ lunch.' or 'your next session will be a practical in…' At the same time, turn off the projector, collect the papers and turn your back on the learners. When the lecturer hovers without a signal the learners are uncertain whether the session has finished or not. It gives a poor impression of the lecture just fading out and can spoil the dynamic effect of a succinct summary and termination.

Having identified the simple framework, it is worth considering the structure of the three or four 15 minute sections. For each there is a separate set of objectives, a separate, and preferably different approach, to dialogue, as well as questions and a summary of that part. The final summary would include the collation of the previous summaries.

The use of the set, dialogue, closure framework provides a useful basis for preparing lectures. There will be a more detailed section on preparation later in the chapter.

HOW SHOULD A LECTURE BE GIVEN?

Using the framework from the previous section, when the lecture is first planned the needs of adult learners must be considered.

GROUP SIZE OF LESS THAN 50

The whole design should be based around interaction for this size of group. Many of the ideas from small group work can be adapted with larger groups. In groups of 15-20, there should be much interaction. However, in a group of 50, the interaction may have to be thought out in greater detail.

A snowball approach works well. A question or problem is posed and each individual is asked to consider the answer. Pairs are than asked to look for differences in their answer and finally, groups of four are asked to come to a consensus. The timing could be 5 minutes as an individual, 5-10 minutes as a pair, 10 minutes as a group of four. Each group of four is asked to contribute an idea or partial answer. These may be summarised on a chalkboard, a white board or by using the overhead projector. The timings may vary according to the complexity of the problem or question. In some cases, it may be only a minute or two in each stage. With experience, it is possible to see when individuals, pairs, or groups have come to a decision. Then you ask each individual or pair to move on to the next stage. Slower groups may have to be chivvied, whilst faster groups may be given a sting in the tail! Clearly, management of both time and group process is required here. Careful preparation and time allocation is essential to enable the session to finish punctually.

Incorporating all likely ingredients for motivation are some key factors listed next. There is the case-based approach in which one identifies a patient with a particular problem and asks what should happen next. This is well suited to adult learners. Immediately, the lecture becomes meaningful because it has become experience-based. The groups answering the question and addressing the problem posed are kept involved. The way their solutions or answers are dealt with gives some feedback and the next section of the lecture should enable them to reflect. All the important ingredients for adult learners have been incorporated, including changes in activity to enhance the learning capacity.

The lecture must be rehearsed to ensure that the intended timings are right. Experience helps in judging the timings for active participation. At first, do not attempt a full participation for the whole hour, use one part until you have more experience and confidence.

GROUP SIZE 50 - 100

It is more likely that seating will be fixed for this group size and audio visual facilities are likely to be more formal. The lighting may be more sophisticated and the room lack outside windows, so that ventilation and heating problems may occur. For prolonged sessions, it is important to know how room temperature and humidity changes during an hour or day. In this environment where more effort is needed to ensure learners remain alert, active involvement becomes more important. The identification of learners' and lecturer's roles has to be more explicit for each section of the lecture. The purposes should be spelled out more clearly using slides or transparencies.

The division of the lecture into four or five sections of less that 15 minutes each assists the participants' learning capacity. If the lecture is immediately after lunch, use shorter sections.

The use of buzz groups is still possible. However, it is unlikely that learners will be able to rearrange their chairs. One way of overcoming this is to arrange for pairs in two successive rows to act as a group. The two in the front row turn around to discuss with those in the row behind. It may be more convenient to use threes for the differences and fours, fives and even sixes for the consensus. There is no unalterable rule that it should be 1, 2, 4 but there must be a plan for enabling the formation of groups. If the first part requires about 5 minutes for individuals, the lecturer can choose the 'pairings' and the formation of the groups.

Another way of breaking the lecture sequence is by giving learners a short time to check and reflect on their notes. If there are any problems they can ask you or their neighbour.

The use of voice and gesticulation demands more attention for this larger group. Some voice projection may be necessary. Voice projection depends on using the resonance in the sinus region and the chest. Shouting will only give the lecturer a sore throat and be seen as aggressive by the learners. Gestures need to be a little larger than usual. Both of these aspects need some preparation and marginal notes to oneself about projection and particular gesticulations to emphasise points. A rehearsal is even more important for this size of group.

It is still appropriate to check understanding by taking questions at the end of the lecture. An alternative approach is to have one or two transparencies with multiple choice questions. The audience is asked to decide which is the best answer, perhaps by a show of hands. If this approach is used regularly with the same group, there is an increased drive for the learners to stay alert so they can answer questions. A brief discussion after the questions enables reflection and leads into the summary followed by an obvious termination.

GROUP SIZE OVER 100

The situation is much more formal and the environment largely pre-set. The seating will be fixed. Although lighting may include daylight with blinds or curtains, it is more likely to be artificial. The blackout is likely to be very dark. The temperature is usually controlled by mechanical ventilation or air conditioning, both noisy. Darkness and a continuous background drone are excellent sleep aids! It is important to know the facilities. For example, how partial lighting is obtained for audience note taking.

The method of role identification is largely determined by the room design. It is necessary to have a formal statement and clearer change in the lecturer's position for role changes and active participation.

Slides or transparencies are almost essential in this more formal explanation of purposes. Using a chalkboard, whiteboard and flip chart are difficult and very large writing or printing will be necessary. All projected and written visual aids must be checked to ensure that they can be read from the back of the room. The dialogue will be more formal. The use of clear enunciation, good projection (a microphone will usually be available) and large gesticulations become the norm. The lecturer must become an actor for this size of group. Rehearsal is essential and should take place in the actual lecture theatre that is to be used.

The use of learner involvement is more difficult but not impossible. The snowball approach is still feasible, but not all the groups will be able to report. The use of questions that are projected may become more important for each section as well as for the final summary. Questions from the audience may identify potential problems but can only be cursory at the end. If difficulty is raised, find out whether it is common by a show of hands and, if so, deal with it. If it is not a general problem, suggest a meeting with the questioner afterwards. The summary must be formal and projected. The termination is formal and explicit.

It is important to remember the needs of adult learners. Using examples and cases help, but the lecture must not become a long sequence of war stories! The comparing of ideas to learners' experience helps. The opportunity to reflect on that experience is essential. Feedback should arise from the questions. Once more, the division of the lecture into four or five sections helps concentration and capacity to learn.

199

WHAT SHOULD I DO DURING MY LECTURE?

Some of the alternatives for the dialogue have been indicated in the section above. Let us look at some variations. In each of these approaches to dialogue, remember:

* Maintain linkages with other parts of the course.
* Maintain continuity.
* Get and give feedback.

Using Slides

The poor use of slides is an unfortunate characteristic of many lectures. The problem is that slides, low lighting, a monotonous voice and a stuffy room create an ideal environment for sleep! Learners must be actively engaged. Therefore, there must be some ambient light so that the audience can see you and you can see them. You may wish to show a slide and ask them questions, instead of telling them all about it. You must summarise what they have said to make the important issues clear. Remember that in some rooms the audience will have difficulty hearing what is said. You may need to repeat the question or comment for people at the back to hear. By the lecturer's continual use of this approach, learners expect to ask and be asked questions about the slides. They become active rather than passive.

The background colour of slides needs careful consideration when using some ambient light. There should be a good contrast between the lettering and the background. Yellow on royal or dark blue works well. Keep the words on a slide to a minimum. Remember key words or phrases are better than complete sentences. Slides that are of the real thing need to be good quality. The use of blank slides (black) can provide useful cues to the lecturer for a question or a change in activity.

You need to ensure that you know your slides thoroughly, that they are all numbered, the right way up and the right way round. This is your responsibility. Avoid using too many. Too many of your own or obscure clinical slides confuse rather than reinforce key issues. Text should be a maximum of 5-7 words per line, and a maximum of 5-7 lines, preferably less.

Questions and Answers

The approach has already been introduced in the last section. Questions are not just fired from the hip; they need carefully preparing.

Simply there are three types of questions:

1. yes/no
2. closed
3. open

A question requiring a 'yes' or 'no' answer does not stretch the learner very much. However, if you have identified a shy member of the audience who lacks confidence, it may help to use this basic type of question to encourage them.

A closed question requires an answer that is specific and correct:

—*Why may the electrical conduction through the heart be blocked?*

The possible answers would be:

- Ischaemic disease
- Drugs
- Trauma
- Abnormal metabolic conditions.

This represents a useful closed question because it enables you to get four people to answer! Normally, a question beginning *'Why'* or *'How'* would be an open question and usually there is no one right answer.

—*'You have just tried unsuccessfully to resuscitate a child. The child's single parent is at work. How would you go about informing the parent of the child's death?'*

Clearly there is not a right answer, although there are approaches that would not be recommended. *(Give time to think out an answer)*

Asking the question is not enough. Be careful how you respond to the answers. You are trying to help people to learn and enhance their confidence. Do not be sarcastic, saying things like 'That is rubbish!' or 'Haven't you read your text book?' Try to help them to a better answer by posing closed questions. If you cannot see a way towards that, then thank them for their answers, and ask whether someone else can suggest an alternative answer. Eventually, take it back to the original learner and ask that individual whether he or she would like to come up with a choice from the alternatives.

A question and answer session is not easy and needs practice. As in the last section, start with small groups in order to practice the techniques. Then graduate to the lecture, first using it for part of a lecture or for particular slides (perhaps distributed through the lecture). Remember, because of the change in roles, you need another 'set-dialogue-closure' in order to prepare in some detail. When you become more confident with the approach you may wish to use it for a whole lecture.

Flip Charts

Flip charts provide a useful tool for recording learners' answers, or building up ideas. The chart can also be used as a means of summarising their answers. You should have planned in advance what you are going to write and the layout. Flip charts have the advantage that it is easy to go backwards to anything that has been previously written. However, if used as a scribbling pad it can confuse the learners. So again, forethought should be given to likely structures or groupings for the information and a layout prepared.

To ensure it can be read at the back of the room you must practise your writing, including its size. This method is most suitable for group sizes of under 50, but may be possible for the 50-100, depending on the room shape and size. It should not be used for larger groups.

Overhead Projector

A slightly more formal lay out for the room is needed with the overhead projector. It is best used with the screen diagonally across one corner of the room, and with the top of the screen leaning forward to get a rectangular image. Make sure the seating positions are arranged so that everyone has an unobstructed view and remember that the presenter may cause some form of obstruction so check the seating positions.

Prepared transparencies are best. Limit the number of lines and words for text slides. As a rough guide:

- Use maximum of 7 lines.
- Use maximum of 5 words on a line.
- Use minimum size of font equal to 1/20 vertical height.

An overhead projector's light level is less powerful than that of a slide projector so it is less satisfactory for colour pictures. It is more flexible than 35mm slides but less than the flip chart because partial blackout may be required on sunny days.

While you can use it for writing in front of the audience, you must practice good writing. It is possible to project computer output.

A modern equivalent uses a rostrum with a TV camera and TV projection. Either printed material or overhead projector type transparencies can be used. All the issues about visibility and contrast apply.

Chalk and Talk

Much that applies to the flip chart also applies to the chalkboard. Writing needs practice. Check that it can be read from the back of the room. A plan needs to be in hand for the board layout, particularly if it is a big one. A good layout helps to pull together and emphasise the key issues. One useful tip is to section off and quarter as a scribbling pad. From this, major points can be taken and given structure on the rest of the board. This allows the board to be used for a lecture that builds up the key issues. The lecturer may talk, use hand outs, use question and answer, but the chalkboard will have the build up of the key issues. Its advantage over any of the previous approaches is that, with good planning, everything can be on the board at the end of the lecture and used for a summary.

Handouts

Handouts are useful for learners writing their own notes, for diagrams, charts, or graphs not in the manual, or for providing a complete set of your notes.

If simply written down verbatim, the latter is not much help to a learner. Your notes should be translated into their own situations by a process of reflection. A better way would be a skeleton of your notes with spaces for them to add their own comments. Handouts may be given before the session as an advanced organiser. These help to ensure a baseline knowledge on which to proceed and should be well constructed, easily read and understood. A handout given at the beginning of a lecture can be a distraction unless the learners have time to read it and are directed as to how it may be used for note-taking.

Yourself

Whether you like it or not you are an essential part of the audio-visual presentation. The way you stand or sit sends immediate messages to those ever inquisitive eyes. A tentative, nervous start worries them too. A confident opening forms the basis for a successful lecture.

There are some useful tips worth remembering:

- Keep it simple.
- Keep eye contact with your audience (scan all of them).
- Do not move about too much.
- Avoid reading notes on slides but use them as triggers for ideas.
- Speak clearly rather than loudly.
- Use silences and pauses.
- Make clear transitions from one part to another.
- Ensure participation.
- Avoid turning your back.

If you are nervous then you might find the following ideas helpful:

- Take one or two deep breaths before you start.
- Tense yourself up all over then relax.
- Know your first few 'lines' off by heart.

If you try to memorise everything the lecture will lack spontaneity and flexibility. Remember and link ideas logically by giving each a set-dialogue-closure format. Mini set-dialogue-closure sequences may comprise a lecture, followed by a demonstration of a skill, followed by a question and answer session

Television

The use of television in lectures can be live or recorded. The use of a live link requires a very confident lecturer and excellent communication with those in the live situation. Recordings enable editing to highlight the key aspects. Also, they enable short sequences followed by questions. Using these shorter sequences is another way of keeping sequences to a maximum of 15 minutes and incorporating changes in activities. The use of sequences can also lead to 'what would you do next?' when something has gone wrong. Perhaps, this is a good use of the snowball approach. The next sequence then shows what actually happened.

Television usually needs dimmed light. Extensive use of TV, especially if it is live, can lead to sleepiness. Surgery, like war, consists of sharp blasts of high activity, punctuating much longer periods of routine, often boredom. Be prepared to liven up the quiet times with questions, discussions, and some work on a flip chart or overhead projector.

HOW SHOULD I PREPARE MY LECTURES?

There are different ways of using lecture notes. The full text type of notes present a variety of problems:

- The written word is used instead of the spoken word (the spoken word uses a vocabulary of about 200-300 words whereas the written word uses at least 2 or 3 thousand).
- It is difficult to find the place once it has been lost.
- It is difficult to get back into the flow when there has been a question or other deviation from the script.

Using cards allows more flexibility. The cards should have key words or phrases to enable easy reference. They can be held together with a tag, to prevent nervous lecturers dropping them into a random order! If detailed notes are needed for a specific part, it is probably better to have them on a separate sheet of paper. The card type of notes also has disadvantages:

- It is difficult to find the place once it has been lost.
- There is no detail of specific parts.

A third alternative is to use mind maps or spider diagrams. Here, the title is placed in the centre. Each main theme is an arm from the centre with subdivisions for each part. Inter connections can be shown by lines outside the diagram. An example would look like:

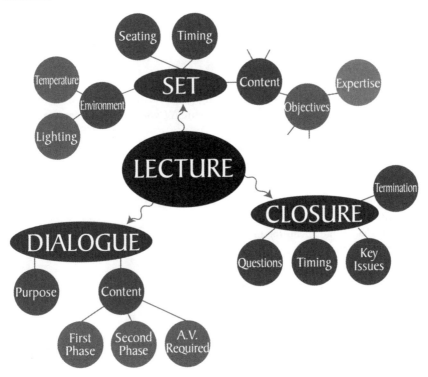

The remaining ends of the lines in the example would be the headings for each section of this chapter. The diagram becomes very specific to an individual's ideas about the subject and, as it deals with concepts, is easy to talk from.

When preparing a lecture, the following skeleton may be helpful:

Objectives

What do you want the learners to learn or do? What competencies should they achieve? How will you know when they have achieved this knowledge or competency? How will you assess it?

State the objectives/competencies that are expected from the lecture as follows:

By the end of the session, the learners will know/understand/be able to do the following.

_____

_____

The more specific the statement, the easier it will be to develop the session.

Teaching approach

Remember that you are trying to enable the learners to learn. You need to think about the sequence (timings), the sort of questions that you will use, how and who among the learners you will involve? How can you check that they value what you are telling them?

Allocate a time for each part of the learning process. For example, in a 15 minute session:

Set	2 minutes
Dialogue	10 minutes
Closure	3 minutes

SET

Think about the seating or standing arrangement for the learners, your role and where you want to stand/sit, what equipment/AV you need, and remember the objectives.

Identify your role relative to the learners. Do you expect them to sit and listen? Do you expect them to interact with you or one another?

_____

_____

Identify chair requirements for an arrangement that allows this interaction or organise the learners in the rows.

_____

_____

Remember the objectives that you stated above.
How long will you need to make the purposes of the session clear to the learners?

_____

_____

DIALOGUE

Think about your beginning statements or questions, what follow-up you will use, timing the parts of this dialogue; rather than just talking to them, try to involve learners and get them to think and reflect.

First phase (duration)

_____

Purpose (what you will tell the learners about this section)

_____
_____

Content

_____
_____

Questions asked or statements made to relate to hospital practice or to the lectures, practicals or clinical sessions in the course.

_____
_____

AV requirements

_____
_____

Questions (allow a short time)
Summary (what you will tell students are the key issues)

_____
_____

Second phase (same aspects as for the first phase, perhaps some humour. Is there a possible change of style to aid attention?)

_____
_____

Third phase (duration, etc.)

_____
_____

CLOSURE

Find out whether learners have any questions. You need to control this, see below.

Pull together in a few simple words, the key issues that have been learned in the session.

List these

_____

_____

Do you need any AV for this?

_____

_____

How much time will you need for this_____(needs to be subtracted from total time available. Care and discipline must be exercised as closures have a habit of dragging or allowing a well planned session to overrun.) Make it clear that you have finished. For example, turn off the projector, collect up your papers and thank them, then tell them to go to the next session.

ANSWERING QUESTIONS

As a general rule give short specific answers. Any attempt at elaboration by them (or you!) should be kept for breaks such as the coffee, lunch.

One or two examples:

Q.   Could you go back through/repeat the explanation of…

A.   Is this a problem for everyone? (If the answer is 'yes', you need to re-explain briefly; if 'no' then offer to see those having difficulties over coffee, lunch, etc.)

Q.   In our hospital/department we…

Beware

A.   I would like to discuss that with you later (e.g. over coffee, lunch, etc.)

Q.   Have you got any references to papers that support this approach?

Beware

A.   Yes (if you have!) I will get a copy sent to all the course participants. If you do not have any idea, ask if any other members of faculty have. If nobody has, then offer to send a paper in due course - or refer to the library.

Q.   What was the name of/the meaning of…

A.   Give a very short answer (Do not digress otherwise you could be into one of the previous questions!)

You may wish to devise an alternative basis for preparation. Remember the key issues of involving, experience, reflection on the experience, feedback and learning capacity. These should be included in the set, dialogue and closure framework.

Rehearsals are essential for the first time. The use of complex audio-visual facilities such as computer controlled projectors, computer generated slides, TV should be rehearsed several times, and there should be alternative approaches ready in case of technical problems.

STUDENT PRESENTATIONS

Students need to have the same guidelines for preparing presentations. The idea of rehearsals is essential for them. The facilities that are to be available should become familiar to minimise problems over the normal nerves of first time presentation.

If hand written transparencies are to be used on the overhead projector, insist on lower case printing with the transparency laid over a sheet of lined paper to provide even lettering. Colours can be useful if they are not over done. For larger groups or presentations of their research, try to make more professional or computer-generating facilities available for transparencies or encourage them to access them elsewhere. There may be computer facilities available on the network to enable them to generate 35mm slides.

SUMMARY

All lectures must be carefully planned, structured and well prepared. This preparation should include a clear idea of the environment and how it will be used. The design of a lecture for adult learners should include the learners being active (mentally!) during the lecture. There should be variation in the type of activity. The goals of the lecture should be clearly stated and, at the outset, any expectation of learner involvement should be made explicit.

The main part of the lecture will involve the lecturer talking, interaction between the lecturer and the learners and, possibly, learner/learner interaction. Remember, it is dialogue, not monologue. Learners should be able to relate content to their and your experience. Any of the learners activities can be made more meaningful through feedback and through enabling them to reflect on the experience. In a one-hour lecture, there should be three or four sections lasting not more than 15 minutes.

Just before the end of the lecture, and possibly at the end of each section, there should be an opportunity for the learners to ask questions. The lecture concludes after a summary of the key issues and the end of the lecture should be clearly signalled.

Lecturers have a responsibility to promote learning through the creation of a planned, informed and well delivered learning exercise. Learners, through motivation and active participation must be helped to relate the content to their own experience.

208

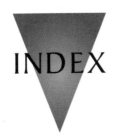

INDEX

211

212

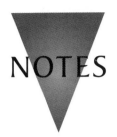

NOTES

213

214